INTERMITTENT FASTING

FOR WOMEN OVER 50

Winning Formula to Reset Your Metabolism, Delay Aging, and Lose Weight With 150+ Healthy Recipes and a Beginner-Proof 21-Day Meal Plan to Regain Your Best Shape

LISA MIDDLETON

Table of Contents

INTRODUCTION

Women over the age of 50 can encounter difficulties while attempting to lose weight. It may be due to a variety of factors. Sometimes, the primary culprit is a slowed metabolism. Your metabolism will be quicker if you have more lean muscle. However, when we age, we eventually lose healthy muscle mass and sometimes will be less active than we were. As a result? Stubborn excess fat accumulates that simply would not budge.

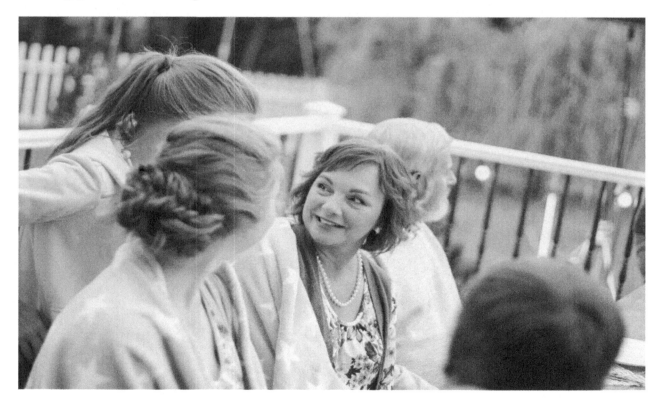

Intermittent fasting has grown in popularity over the last few years due to the variety of health benefits and the fact that it does not limit food options. Unlike other diets, which dictate when you should eat, intermittent fasting emphasizes what you should eat by adding daily short-term fasts into your schedule. This eating plan may assist you in consuming fewer calories, losing weight, and decreasing the risk of developing heart disease or diabetes.

Intermittent fasting can aid in weight loss and reduce the risk of developing age-related illnesses in women over 50.

Several factors contribute to losing weight after the age of 50, including a slower metabolism, achy muscles, decreased muscle mass, and sleep problems. Simultaneously, losing weight, including dangerous belly fat, will significantly lower the risk of developing severe health problems such as diabetes, cancer and heart attacks.

Naturally, as you age, the chance of contracting a variety of diseases increases. In certain cases, IF for women over 50 can act as a modern fountain of youth in weight loss and reduce the risk of developing age-related ailments.

Fasting has been shown to increase metabolism, mental wellbeing and can also help combat some cancers. Additionally, it can help women over 50 avoid some muscle, joint and nerve conditions.

Several reports, however, have shown that intermittent fasting might not be as helpful to women as it is to men. Thus, it may be important for women to adopt a modified method.

Here is a comprehensive introduction to intermittent fasting for women over 50.

Chapter 1.

WHAT IS INTERMITTENT FASTING?

Intermittent fasting is not really a diet but just a way of eating. It is a method of planning your meals, so you get the best out of them. Intermittent fasting does not modify what you eat; rather, it adjusts when you eat.

Intermittent fasting requires that you consume food only within a specified period. Fasting for a set number of hours per day or consuming just one meal a few days a week will make your body lose fat. Furthermore, scientific research suggests that there might be certain health advantages.

Mark Mattson, Ph.D., a neuroscientist at Johns Hopkins, has been researching intermittent fasting for around 25 years. He claims that our bodies have developed to go without food for several hours, days, or even weeks. Before humans began farming, they were hunter-gatherers who adapted to survive — and grow — for prolonged periods without eating. They had no choice but to Hunting games, and gathering nuts and berries required a lot of time and effort.

It was easier to keep a healthier weight even 50 years ago. Christie Williams, M.S., R.D.N., a dietitian at Johns Hopkins, explains: "There were no devices, and T.V. programs were switched off at 11 p.m.; people avoided eating before they went to bed." The portions were much small. More people played and worked outdoors, and they got more exercise in general."

Nowadays, television, the internet, and other types of entertainment are available 24 hours a day, seven days a week. We stay up late to watch our favorite movies, play games and talk online. We spend the whole day — and most of the night — sitting and snacking."

Increased calorie intake and decreased physical exercise will trigger the onset of obesity, type 2 diabetes, heart disease, and other illnesses. According to scientific evidence, intermittent fasting can help mitigate these trends.

Why is it advisable to alter your dietary habits?

Most importantly, it is smart to get slim without being on a fad diet or cutting the calories to nothing. When you first begin intermittent fasting, you will most likely attempt to maintain your calorie intake at the same level. (Most people consume larger portions in a short span of time.) Intermittent fasting is also a healthy way to maintain muscle density when losing fat.

Having said that, the biggest reason people pursue intermittent fasting is to lose weight.

Intermittent fasting is one of the best methods for losing weight and maintaining a healthy weight since it needs relatively little behavioral adjustment. It is a positive idea because it means intermittent fasting is "simple enough that you'll do it, however significant enough that it will really make a difference."

1.1. The Science behind Intermittent Fasting

Intermittent fasting seems to have a wide range of health effects. These results may potentially occur as a result of a metabolic switch being activated.

"Fasting causes a decrease in glucose [blood sugar] levels. As a result, the body switches from glucose to fat as an energy source, after converting the fat to ketones, "describes Kathy McManus, a registered dietitian and head of the Nutrition Department at Harvard-affiliated Women's Hospital. This shift from glucose to ketones as an energy supply alters the body's chemistry in positive ways.

Fasting regularly in animals is correlated with weight reduction and reduced heart rate and blood pressure, decreased insulin tolerance, low "bad" LDL cholesterol levels, high "good" HDL cholesterol levels, and much less inflammation. Few studies have also reported better memory.

Intermittent fasting has also been linked to a longer life period in animals. Why is this so? According to recent Harvard studies, intermittent fasting can allow each cell membrane mitochondria (energy-producing engines) to generate energy more efficiently and stay in a more youthful condition.

"As eating during the day, you are not confronting the mitochondria at night because they should be doing other things," says Dr. William Mair, a physician, and professor of genetics and chronic diseases.

There is also a case of your body's processing of HGH. Our bodies spontaneously generate insulin when we feed in order to conserve glucose from carbs for later usage. We live in a world where most of our meals are routine, and we are constantly bombarded with high fat and sugar ratios in most consumables. It places us in an anabolic state, which means we are continuously gaining weight. Food glucose is retained as fat, resulting in weight gain. Intermittent fasting effectively reverses this mechanism, allowing our cells to use the glucose that has been stored for energy. Weight loss occurs as cells reach a catabolic state (break down). Since HGH is created in response to the body's need for glucose, HGH production is reduced when we receive glucose from somewhere else while we are continuously consuming. HGH oversees controlling metabolism and has a plethora of beneficial properties for muscle regeneration and fat burning. Intermittent fasting has been shown to increase HGH output up to 5 times.

Fasting causes our bodies to enter a slightly stressed state known as hormesis. Our cells evolve during hormesis, which may improve fat burning, metabolic rate, and other internal processes.

Much of the time, athletes consume fewer total calories than non-fasters, resulting in weight loss. It could be attributed to various behavioral causes, or it could be that having a limited window of time for consumption discourages such behaviors, such as late-night snacking.

1.2. How Does Intermittent Fasting Work?

Intermittent fasting can be done in various ways, but they all rely on selecting daily times to eat and fast. For example, you could try eating just eight hours a day and fasting the rest of the time. You may still opt to eat just one meal a day, two days a week. There are several intermittent fasting schedules to choose from.

According to Mattson, after many hours without calories, the body depletes its sugar reserves and begins to burn fat. It is referred to as metabolic switching by him.

"Intermittent fasting conflicts with the typical feeding schedule for most Westerners, who eat throughout the day," Mattson adds. "If somebody eats three meals a day with desserts and snacks and does not exercise, they are consuming a limited number of calories and not losing their fat reserves every time they eat."

Simply put, when readily available glucose is depleted, our insulin levels fall, and our fat cells release their accumulated sugar to be used as energy. This method can help with cellular repair as well as weight loss. In addition, studies have shown that intermittent fasting involves reduced muscle loss than the more traditional form of constant calorie restriction.

Many people feel that IF has helped them mainly because the narrow eating window forces them to consume fewer calories. For example, instead of consuming three meals and two snacks, they realize that they can only have two meals and one snack in the given window. They become more conscious about the foods they eat and prefer to avoid empty calories from carbohydrates and saturated fat.

Naturally, you can also select the types of nutritious foods that appeal to you. While some people use intermittent fasting to limit their total calorie consumption, others pair it with a vegan, keto, or other types of diet.

1.3. Three Significant Advantages and Disadvantages of Intermittent Fasting

Intermittent fasting, the current lifestyle movement that involves not eating at all for short amounts of time, has its advantages and disadvantages, much as anything else.

Intermittent fasting improves body composition, reduces the risk of cancer, and can improve cognitive function.

Among the disadvantages of intermittent fasting are that it may be difficult to maintain over time, can impact your social life, and can result in certain health problems.

It is almost impossible to study dieting or exercise patterns without encountering THE knowledge on intermittent fasting.

The IF trend requires fasting for a specified amount of time without eating any calories, but one key point to remember about fasting is that it can be implemented in various forms.

Some suggest a 16:8 ratio, in which you abstain from food for 16 hours of the day and only eat all your calories and meals for the day during a fixed eight-hour span. Some advocate for 5:2, which entails fasting and eating about 500 calories on two straight days, followed by eating anything you want on the other 5 days of a week. Other ways of extended fasting advocate for a weekly 36-hour fast.

The benefit of intermittent fasting is that its many variants help you choose what works best for you. And, as in anything, there are advantages and disadvantages.

Advantage 1

Intermittent fasting has been shown to boost body composition.

Since you are not consuming calories when fasting, it makes sense to believe that eating less than you usually would result in weight loss. Fasting enables you to burn out all your remaining sugars and then dig through your fat reserves. We continue to lose body fat as we start to burn fat reserves.

According to Healthline, intermittent fasting improves body composition by allowing less food intake, encouraging weight reduction and reduced body fat, and altering our metabolism by its hormonal impact.

Disadvantage 1

It may be challenging to maintain a long-term commitment.

Intermittent fasting means that you fast for a predetermined amount of time, then consume a predetermined number of calories during a predetermined window of time, then reverse to establish a caloric deficit. This extended duration of calorie deprivation can be challenging to maintain long-term thanks to low energy, cravings, routines, and the consistency needed to adhere to the time frames accompanying your intermittent fasting times.

Intermittent fasting is often difficult to maintain over time due to the level of self-control involved. Both aspects of intermittent fasting may be challenging; avoiding food while you should be fasting and not overeating when it is time to eat are critical.

Brad Pilon, author and researcher of a famous book on Intermittent Fasting, says that "once your fast is complete, you must pretend that it never happened." There is no reimbursement, no bonus, no special diet, no unique shakes, beverages, or tablets."

Although this can be challenging, it is essential for the process and, consequently, for you to gain intermittent fasting.

Advantage 2

Intermittent fasting can aid in preventing and reducing the risk of disease.

According to Express, intermittent fasting has the potential to "have a positive effect on certain critical risk markers for cardiovascular disease."

According to the Cleveland Clinic, fasting can aid in regulating diabetes, cholesterol, and blood pressure, all of which are critical factors that should be monitored for disease prevention.

According to a study conducted by scientists at the University of Surrey, individuals who adopted an intermittent fasting diet saw a 9% decrease in blood pressure compared to a 2%

rise in those who practiced a more conventional, regular diet.

Another research discovered intermittent fasting improved sleep time, which reduces blood sugar and inflammation, two major risk factors for serious diseases such as diabetes or heart diseases.

Disadvantage 2

It can harm your social life.

Let us face it, most of our social experiences revolve around food and beverages. When fasting, you must either have the courage to refrain from indulging or devise ways to maintain a social life until breaking your fast.

Though challenging, it is feasible.

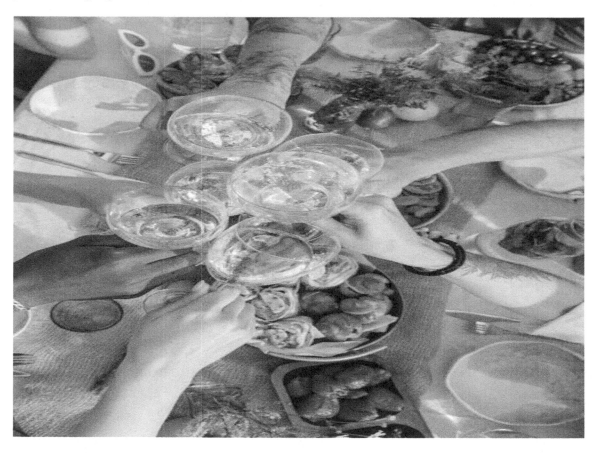

Fasting can be stressful, though. During the fasting periods, you may have reduced levels of energy than normal and might feel unable to get out and about or as though you just need to relax and save the energy you do have.

It is a tough balancing act.

Advantage 3

Intermittent fasting encourages healthy brain activity.

It will assist the brain in functioning more efficiently.

Fasting accelerates neurogenesis in the brain, described as "the growth and production of new nerve tissues and brain cells," explains a professor of neurology, improving cognitive capacity, mood, concentration, and memory.

Moreover, Mattson states that abstaining from eating places pressure on the brain, prompting it to take preventative action against diseases. It is due to the body entering ketosis, a metabolic state in which fat is used as a fuel supply to "improve vitality and eliminate brain fog."

We have already learned that puzzles and other cognitively challenging activities are beneficial, and it appears that the difficulties associated with fasting are as well.

Disadvantages 3

There is an increased chance of developing certain adverse health effects. Your body may become susceptible to health problems. Individuals who already lead an active lifestyle or are leaner prior to starting intermittent fasting can experience hormonal imbalances consequently.

It may result in erratic menstrual periods and the possibility of fertility problems in females. Hormonal imbalances may result in insomnia, elevated stress, or thyroid problems in everyone.

Intermittent fasting is relatively appropriate for most people when done under the guidance or consent of a practitioner and with proper observation of bodily functions.

Chapter 2.

INTERMITTENT FASTING IN WOMEN

Intermittent Fasting (IF) is quickly becoming one of the most effective methods for losing weight, becoming lean, and getting fit. Intermittent fasting for males and females has gradually gained traction as more people became conscious of the benefits.

According to studies, intermittent fasting does more than just burn fat. According to Mattson, "as modifications arise in this metabolic switch, it impacts the brain and body."

One of Mattson's findings, reported in the British Medical Journal, revealed information regarding various health advantages correlated with the discipline. All involve a longer lifespan, a leaner frame, and a clearer mind.

"Some things happen through intermittent fasting that may defend organs from chronic diseases like a coronary failure, age-related neurodegenerative conditions, type 2 diabetes, including inflammatory intestinal disease and many cancers," he adds.

Intermittent fasting boosts strength and energy levels. Best of all, the outcomes keep you going. It is often claimed to increase cognitive function. However, since the procedure is not suitable for all, many people remain wary of its efficacy.

While shorter fasting times are assumed healthy for many folks, longer ones are not advised for certain women.

2.1. Men and Women Can Be Affected Differently by Intermittent Fasting

There has been some suggestion that intermittent fasting might not be as effective for some females as males.

According to one report, blood sugar balance worsened in women after 21 days of intermittent fasting, but not in men.

There are also several anecdotal accounts about women who witnessed shifts in their menstrual periods since beginning Intermittent Fasting. Such changes may arise as female bodies are particularly vulnerable to calorie restriction.

When calorie consumption is limited, like when fasting for an extended period or fasting regularly, a small brain area known as the hypothalamus is influenced.

It can interfere with the release of GnRH (gonadotropin-releasing hormone), a hormone that aids in the secretion of two reproductive hormones: follicle-stimulating hormone (F.S.H.) and luteinizing hormone (L.H.).

If these hormones are unable to interact with the ovaries, females run a risk of irregular cycles, miscarriage, low bone health, and other health issues.

While no comparative human trials have been conducted, experiments in rats have shown that 3–6 months of alternate-day fasting triggered a decrease in ovary size and abnormal reproductive system in female rats.

For these considerations, women should take a modified strategy to intermittent fasting. Fasting for a shorter time and having fewer fasting days have shown greater results in women's health and wellbeing.

2.2. Women's Benefits of Intermittent Fasting Can Extend Past Calorie Restriction

Many nutritionists believe that IF only succeeds as it automatically reduces their food consumption, but others differ. They claim that intermittent fasting produces greater outcomes than traditional meal plans containing the same number of calories as well as other nutrients. Many studies also indicate that fasting for several hours each day does more than just reduce the number of calories consumed.

Here are several **metabolic improvements** caused by IF that can help explain synergistic benefits:

HGH: As insulin levels fall, HGH levels increase, promoting fat burning as well as muscle development.

Noradrenaline: In reaction to an empty stomach, the nervous system sends this chemical to cells to inform them that they must release fat for energy.

More Health Advantages

Several animal and human research indicate that intermittent fasting can provide additional health benefits.

Reduced inflammation: According to some reports, intermittent fasting may minimize the main markers of inflammation. Chronic inflammation may result in weight gain and various health issues.

Psychological wellbeing: In one research, seven weeks of intermittent fasting reduced stress and excessive eating while raising body confidence in obese adults.

Maintain muscle mass: Unlike constant calorie restriction, intermittent fasting tends to be more successful at maintaining muscle mass. Increased muscle mass allows you to eat more calories and rest.

Cell Reparation: Since the body is not focused on digestion, the healing mechanism is in full swing. It will fully focus on cell repair. This is known as autophagy. Thus, fasting aids in the healing or, in this situation, restoration of the body and its correct functioning.

Improves clarity of thought: Another significant advantage to intermittent fasting is that it allows you to concentrate better on tasks and fulfill a significant portion of the job while fasting.

Prevention of Insulin tolerance: Insulin tolerance develops when the blood sugar levels are consistently high. As a result, the body cannot function on and break down the sugar content of your blood. Intermittent fasting allows you to maintain your blood sugar levels in balance. This disease may also be caused by high blood pressure, sedentary behavior, genes, poor diet, obesity, or an excess of body weight.

Insulin is a hormone that regulates blood sugar levels. Lower insulin levels during the fasting cycle can aid in fat burning. Intermittent fasting is not only good for the waistline, but it can also reduce your chances of contracting a variety of chronic diseases.

Cardiovascular Protection: Heart disease is the primary cause of mortality on a global scale. Elevated blood pressure, high LDL cholesterol, and high triglyceride levels are also contributing factors for the occurrence of cardiac disease.

In one trial of 16 obese women and men, intermittent fasting reduced blood pressure by 7% in only eight weeks. The same research discovered intermittent fasting reduced LDL cholesterol by 24% and triglycerides by 31%.

The evidence for a correlation between intermittent fasting and lower triglyceride levels, on the other hand, is inconsistent.

A survey of 40 people of average weight showed that four weeks of prolonged fasting over the Islamic holiday of Ramadan had little effect on triglycerides or LDL cholesterol. Until researchers properly explain the impact of intermittent fasting on cardiac health, higher-quality trials with more rigorous methods are needed.

Diabetes: Intermittent fasting will also help you control and lower the risk of type 2 diabetes. Intermittent fasting, including prolonged calorie restriction, serves to decrease some of the risk indicators for diabetes. It accomplishes this mostly by reducing insulin levels and decreasing insulin tolerance.

Six months of intermittent fasting cut insulin levels by 28% and insulin tolerance by 18% in a randomized controlled trial of more than 100 overweight or obese women. Blood sugar levels stayed constant.

Furthermore, 8–14 weeks of intermittent fasting has been found to reduce insulin levels by 21–30% and blood glucose levels by 4–7% in people with pre-diabetes, a disease in which blood glucose levels are elevated but not severe enough to diagnose diabetes.

In terms of blood sugar, though, intermittent fasting might not be as effective for females as males. A limited study showed that after 22 days of alternate day fasting, women's blood sugar management deteriorated, while men's blood sugar had a little detrimental impact. Despite this side effect, the decrease in insulin and insulin tolerance will also lower the risk of diabetes, particularly in pre-diabetics.

Weight Reduction: When performed correctly, intermittent fasting can be an easy and efficient way to reduce weight since brief daily fasts can help you eat fewer calories and drop pounds.

Several reports indicate that intermittent fasting is almost as successful as conventional calorie-restricted diets for short-term weight reduction. A 2018 study of trials of overweight adults discovered that intermittent fasting resulted in an overall weight reduction of 17 lbs. (7.5 kg) over 3 to–12 months.

Another study found intermittent fasting decreased body weight by 4–9 percent in obese or overweight individuals over 4–24 weeks. The review also discovered that participants cut their waist circumference by 4–7% during the same period.

It should be remembered that the long-term implications of intermittent fasting on female weight loss are uncertain. Intermittent fasting in women seems to help with weight reduction in the short term. The amount you lose, though, will most definitely be determined by the number of calories you eat during non-fasting hours and how long you stick to the lifestyle.

Switching to intermittent fasting may help you eat less naturally. According to one report, when the food consumption was limited to a four-hour duration for an individual, they consumed 650 fewer calories per day.

Another research looked at the impact of a lengthy, 36-hour fast on the eating patterns of 24 active men and women. Despite eating more calories on the post-fast day, subjects reduced their overall calorie intake by 1,900 calories, a substantial decrease.

Chapter 3.

WHY DO YOU NEED IF DIET AFTER 50?

Women are usually pre- and post-menopausal at this age, with the average time of menopause being 53. A change usually follows it in body fat distribution from the thighs and hips to the lower belly. Women weaken their defense against osteoporosis and heart disease and as their estrogen levels drop. Intermittent fasting can assist with going through weight gain from menopause, as well as lowering blood cholesterol, blood pressure, insulin resistance, and improving sleep.

Unlike typical food diets, Intermittent Fasting promotes weight loss by restricting food consumption within fasting periods, reducing snacking. A structured process eliminates other unhealthy eating habits that lead to digestion problems and weight fluctuations. But apart from weight loss, intermittent fasting (IF) has a plethora of possible health effects due to natural improvements in bodily processes.

While this cohort has not been specifically analyzed, many of the studies mentioned above had women over the age of 50 in their data analysis.

3.1. Lose the Belly.

The first of their findings from the study mentioned above was that fasting was effective in helping females lose belly fat. Many post-menopausal women are concerned with their belly fat, not just for beauty but also for their welfare.

The women's risk of metabolic syndrome was reduced due to the decrease of belly fat caused by intermittent fasting. A metabolic syndrome is a group of health conditions that raise a post-menopausal woman's diabetes and cardiovascular disease risk.

3.2. Longevity

One part of intermittent fasting that is intriguing and ground-breaking is its anti-aging results and its advances in terms of lifespan. According to a study released in Cell in December 2015, calorie restriction may delay aging. According to a Harvard study, IF can change the role of mitochondria (power-producing systems in cells) and potentially prolong life spans. Fasting can activate mitochondrial networks, keeping them young and promoting fat metabolism. Autophagy is largely accomplished by the body's normal process of removing all defective cells and replacing them with new healthy ones. It is like recycling. It is very promising in terms of long-term viability. A healthy and natural method of replacing old cells and turning back the clock by creating new cells.

Autophagy has been hardwired into us by our ancestors and serves to complement the body's energy supply (self-eating). Of course, this cannot be sustained indefinitely, but the body does not want this to continue indefinitely because you will be feeding every day. When our cells get nervous, intermittent fasting increases autophagy. Autophagy is activated to help preserve and replenish the body. It literally lengthens our life; the test ideas on rats are astounding, showing that calorie restriction increases rats' lives by 31%. No medications, no drugs, just a simple trick that we can all use in our daily lives.

3.3. Joint Well-being

According to the researchers, fasting has increased muscle and joint health, so arthritic symptoms and low back pain were less severe. And a couple of the experiments they looked at found that fasting changed how your body develops hormones that control bone minerals, including phosphate and calcium, so there was some evidence linking fasting to better bone health.

3.4. Cancer

Fasting over varying periods of time helps middle-aged women decrease their risk of major diseases, with much of the literature focusing on the beneficial impact fasting had on cancer. According to the report, fasting seems to block some of the mechanisms contributing to cancer and may also delay tumor development.

3.5. Brain health

According to scientific evidence, IF can enhance cognitive performance in the brain by decreasing inflammation and the chances of neurological disorders (such as Parkinson's). The review report also considered mental health factors, highlighting several findings demonstrating that women who followed various fasting strategies saw improvements in their self-esteem and moods d as well as a decline in depression and anxiety.

3.6. Reduces Insulin Levels

Over time, IF reduces insulin levels in the body, which increases HGH (human growth hormone), which is responsible for the formation and maintenance of healthy tissues. Furthermore, researchers have looked at the beneficial impact of IF on insulin tolerance and lower blood sugar levels, which can help prevent type 2 diabetes.

3.7. Fat-burning and noradrenaline

Fasting stimulates the nervous system to send neurotransmitter signals (noradrenaline) that cause the body to burn fat for fuel.

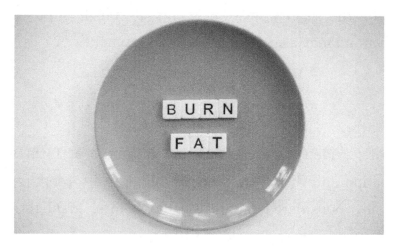

The procedure results in long-term weight loss without sacrificing muscle mass.

3.8. Shield Against Oxidative Stress

Oxidative stress (means unstable molecules that harm cells) plays a part in the growth of a wide range of age-related diseases. According to research, IF will help you boost your biological protection against free radicals and improve your cerebrovascular and cardiovascular fitness.

3.9. Reduces Blood Pressure

High blood pressure has been reported as a potential source of heart disease. Fasting has been shown in studies to boost the protection of your veins and arteries, with a reduction in LDL triglycerides (fat in the bloodstream) and cholesterol.

3.10. Boost Weight Loss

According to a study published in Global Obesity Reports in June 2017, most of the literature on IF has confirmed its contribution to weight loss, with evidence indicating that it can result in a 5 to 9.9 percent reduction in body weight.

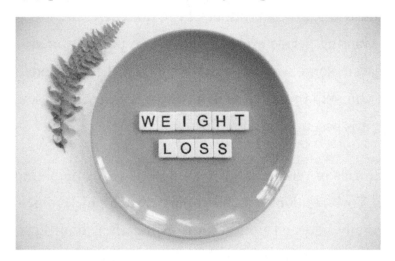

According to a 2018 report published in Diet and Healthy Aging, alternate-day fasting may result in greater fat loss than time-restricted feeding. Still, it may be more difficult to maintain than time-restricted eating. Eventually, further research is required to determine if I.F. will result in actual, long-term weight loss.

3.11. Lower Insulin Resistance

According to a study released in Frontiers of Medicine in February 2014, this disease is a symptom of type 2 diabetes, and being obese raises the risk of insulin resistance. According to a study issued in Nutrients in April 2018, IF can assist with insulin tolerance by lowering total calorie consumption.

3.12. Improved Cardiovascular Well-being

According to a study released in Nutrition Journal, Intermittent Fasting helped study participants reduce weight, fat, and cholesterol levels, prompting researchers to believe that eating this way could help people reduce their chance of coronary heart disease.

3.13. Enhance Metabolic Parameters

All the improved metabolic parameters that we achieve through intermittent fasting all lead to weight loss. Irrespective of losing weight, you can get lower fasting blood glucose, less belly (abdominal) fat, lower blood sugar, triglycerides, and all those things. It has been shown in a few animal trials, but "a number of the qualities that you would physiologically expect from a longer fasting period are not showing in population studies. Also, according to the Nutrients research, some women may have changed their menstrual cycle because of calorie restriction. If you skip three cycles in a row, it is essential to see a doctor; If you skip three cycles in a row, it is essential to see a doctor.

3.14. Stories of Women Above the Age Of 50 Participating In IF

Tris Ford, 54, a New York resident, has been participating in IF since 2016. She only eats one meal a day, normally between 12 and 3:00 in the afternoon. Liza has sustained a 26-pound weight loss since starting IF in 2016. Trish's lupus-related debilitating pain and exhaustion have been relieved by IF. Tris says, "Intermittent fasting has enhanced my understanding of emotional and binge eating, and now I eat intuitively." Trish's most difficult task was getting through breakfast. She got through it by drinking coffee and gradually lessening the amount of cream she used to zero.

Sam Roy, 56, began IF in 2015 to cure prediabetes and lose weight. She eats according to a 20:4 or 18:6 plan. She has managed a 25-pound weight loss since 2015. "I love the fasting phase," Sam says. "IF feels quite natural, and I never have hunger pangs or cravings." Sam also leads an extremely healthy lifestyle, walking daily while fasting with no efficiency or energy problems. "During my workouts, my body has been conditioned to use renewable sources of energy."

Chapter 4.

TYPES OF INTERMITTENT FASTING

As the name implies, intermittent fasting is fasting for a specified period, usually between 12 and 48 hours. The period is referred to as the 'fasting window' during which coffee, water, and herbal tea are allowed, and bone broth is also permitted in some cases. During fasting times, it is advised to take supplements and drink juices prepared from low-calorie veggies. It maintains consistent vitamin and mineral levels.

Following the fasting window, there is a feeding window. This window is usually between 6 and 12 hours long. The fasting and feeding windows will vary since there are many IF processes, one of which is more extreme than the others.

It would help if you worked with them to determine which approach is the right fit for you and your lifestyle. There are several variations of this eating trend. Each approach has the potential to be reliable but determining which one is the most efficient is subjective.

The following are the 10 popular methods of intermittent fasting.

4.1. The 16/8 Technique

How: Fasting for 16 hours and eating for 8 hours.

The 16/8 process entails fasting for 14–16 hrs. per day and limiting your feeding duration to 8–10 hrs. It is entirely up to you to choose which 16 hours of the 24 you want to fast. You

may select an eating time of 7 a.m. to 3 p.m., 11 a.m. to 7 p.m., or noon to 8 p.m., if it is 16 hours of uninterrupted fasting. You can eat 2, 3, or 4 meals during the feeding window.

Fasting this way can be as easy as abstaining from food after dinner and avoiding breakfast. Most people who commit to this plan prefer to miss breakfast instead of dinner, but everyone's life rhythm is unique.

What is best about this plan that you will sleep at least 7-8 of those 16 hours, so we are only just fasting for about 9-8 hours a day. Besides this, we think the Intermittent Fasting 16/8 approach is the most efficient and simplest to begin with. For instance, if you end your dinner at 8 p.m. and do not eat again before noon the following day, you are practically fasting for 16 hours.

Women are usually advised to fast for 14–15 hours as they seem to do best with significantly shorter fasts. This technique, dubbed the Leangains protocol, was popularized by fitness expert Martin Berkhan. This approach can take some time to adjust to those who are particularly hungry and enjoy eating breakfast. Nevertheless, many breakfast skippers eat this way instinctively.

You can drink water, coffee, or other zero-calorie drinks during the fast, which can help alleviate hunger pangs. It is important to focus on consuming nutritious foods during your eating

periods. This process will not work if you consume an unhealthy amount of fast food or calories.

4.2. The 18/6 Technique

How: Fasting for 18 hours and eating for 6 hours.

Very similar to the previous method, the 18/6 Intermittent Fasting Plan requires you to fast for 18 hours and eat within a 6-hour timeframe. It is only two additional hours of fasting per day, but those two hours can make a lot of difference for a beginner faster. That is why we suggest beginning with the 16/8 approach for at least a month before progressing to 18/6 so that you can have a far more satisfying start, which is a critical factor in deciding whether to leave.

Slow but steady wins the race – ease up and pay attention to your body before pushing yourself to the limit.

4.3. The 5:2 Technique A.K.A. The Fast Diet

How: Two days a week, limit calories to 500-600, and five days a week, consume normally.

The 5:2 diet requires you to normally eat five days a week and restrict your calorie consumption to 500–600 calories on the remaining two days. When choosing the fasting days, bear in mind that they should be separated by at least one day of normal feeding. Women should consume 500 calories, and men should consume 600.

For instance, you can normally eat on all days except for Mondays and Thursdays. You consume two small meals per day of 250 calories each for women and 300 calories each for men during those two days. Often known as the Fast Diet, this diet was popularized by British journalist Michael Mosley.

Please keep in mind that the results are entirely dependent on what you eat over the five days of non-fasting; thus, maintain a healthy and balanced diet throughout to achieve the best results. As skeptics point out, no trials are examining the 5:2 diet specifically, but many studies examine the advantages of intermittent fasting.

4.4. The 24-Hour Fast A. K. A. Eat Stop Eat

How: fasting for 24 hours, 1-2 days a week.

Eat Stop Eat entails a once- or twice-weekly 24-hour fast. When fasting for 24 hours, you can reduce the average calorie consumption by approximately 10%, thereby losing weight.

By fasting from dinner to dinner the following day, equates to a complete 24-hour fast. For instance, if you complete dinner at 8 p.m. on Monday and do not eat again until 8 p.m. on Tuesday, you have achieved a complete 24-hour fast. You may also fast between breakfasts or lunches — the outcome is the same.

During the fast, water, coffee, and other zero-calorie drinks are permitted, but no solid foods are allowed. If you are attempting to reduce weight, it is imperative that you consume regular quantities of food during the feeding hours. In other words, you must eat as well as you would if you had not been fasting at all.

The theoretical disadvantage of this approach is that a true 24-hour fast can be very challenging for many people. However, you do not need to go all-in immediately. It is acceptable to begin with 14–16 hours and gradually increase. This technique was popularized by fitness specialist Brad Pilon and has maintained a high level of popularity for many years.

4.5. The 20/4 Technique A. K. A. Warrior Diet

How: Fasting for 20 hours and then eating for 4 hours.

Compared to other approaches, the 20/4 Intermittent Fasting Schedule allows for consuming vegetables and raw fruits and lean protein over the 20-hour fast time. It entails snacking on veggies and raw fruits during the day and indulging in a large meal at night. Essentially, you fast through the day and feed during a four-hour feeding time at night.

This fasting regimen is focused on assuming that our forefathers spent their days harvesting and hunting and only feasted at night. As a result, the 4-hour feeding window should be in the evening, and you should consume food classes in a specific order: greens first, followed by fats and protein, and carbs only if you still feel hungry.

The food preferences on this diet are very similar to those on the paleolithic diet — primarily whole, natural foods. This Warrior Diet was among the first mainstream diets to incorporate some form of intermittent fasting. Ori Hofmekler, a fitness pioneer, popularized the Warrior Diet.

4.6. The 23/1 Technique A. K. A. OMAD Fasting (One Meal A Day)

How: Fasting for 23 hours and then eating just once a day.

Another famous fasting plan is the one-meal-a-day diet (OMAD). And it is exactly how it sounds – just pick a time of the day that is most convenient for you to eat your one and sole meal of the day.

I hear what you are saying – is not that on the verge of starvation? And you are right – the OMAD plan cannot be followed without considering how to consume at least 1200 calories during a single meal. Thus, if you want to fast on 23/1, ensure that your meal is substantial and nutritious.

4.7. Fasting on Alternate Days

How: Alternate-day fasting is when you abstain from food on alternate days.

This method is available in a variety of variations. Several of them make approximately 500 calories on fasting days.

Numerous in vitro trials demonstrating the health effects of intermittent fasting used a variation of this process.

A complete fast any other day can seem excessive and is therefore not suggested for beginners. This approach will cause you to go to bed extremely hungry many days a week, which is unpleasant and potentially undesirable in the long run.

4.8. Spontaneous Meal Skipping

How: Skip a meal when you do not feel like eating

You may not have to pursue a formal intermittent fasting regimen to reap any of the advantages of intermittent fasting. Another choice is to miss meals on occasion, for example, when you are not hungry or are too occupied with preparing and eating. It is a misconception that people must consume food every few hours to avoid going into hunger mode or losing muscle. Your body is well-equipped to withstand prolonged periods of starvation, let alone skipping one or two meals.

Thus, if you are truly not hungry on a particular day, miss breakfast in favor of a nutritious lunch and dinner. Alternatively, if you are traveling and cannot find something you want to eat, consider doing a short fast. When you feel compelled to do so, skipping one or two mealtimes is essentially a random spontaneous fast. Simply ensure that you consume nutritious foods at all your meals.

4.9. Circadian Rhythm Fasting

How: Begin fasting when the sun sets and resume eating when the sun rises.

You may have learned that our bodies are programmed to operate on a Circadian schedule – an inside clock that operates 24 hours a day and controls our energy levels according to the day and night cycle. Thus, if you fast according to the Circadian Rhythm, you will cause daylight to dictate your hours.

Your feeding window begins with the sun rising. If the sun has set and it becomes dark, you can begin your fast. The only disadvantage is that its performance is highly location-dependent. For 76 days, the sun does not set, and it is a fasting time that we strongly advise against in northern Norway.

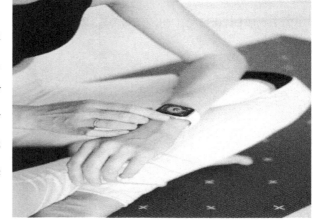

4.10. Prolonged A.K.A. Extended Fasting

How: Once a month, fast for more than 24 hours.

As previously said, prolonged or extended fasting usually refers to a period lasting between 24 and 86 hours without food. It is not advisable to do this fast more than once a month, and any fast longer than 48-72 hours should be performed under the supervision of a physician.

Although many people disregard this suggestion and nothing happens, but it is dangerous, and we do not advise it if you are inexperienced or have any of the medical conditions.

Chapter 5.

BEST TYPES OF INTERMITTENT FASTING FOR WOMEN

There is no versatile solution to dieting. This saying holds true with intermittent fasting as well. Women, on average, can take a more casual attitude to intermittent fasting than men. It would include shorter fasting times, fewer fasting days, or calorie restriction on fasting days.

The below are a few of the most beneficial forms of Intermittent Fasting (I.F.) for women:

Crescendo Approach: It includes fasting for 12 to 16 hours twice or three times a week. The fasting days should not be simultaneous and should be spread equally across the week (Monday, Wednesday, and Friday).

Eat-stop-eat (or 24-hour protocol): Once or twice a week, a 24-hour complete fast (maximum of two times a week for women). Begin with 14–16 hour fasts and steadily increase the duration.

The 5:2 Diet (or "The Fast Diet"): For two days a week, restrict calories to 25% of your regular diet (about 500 calories) and eat regularly for the remaining five days. Allow one day of normal eating between each fasting day.

Modified Alternative Day Fasting: Fasting every second day but eating "normally" on days without fast. You can eat 20–25 percent of your normal calorie intake (approximately 500 calories) when fasting.

The 16/8 Approach (or the "Leangains method"): involves fasting for 16 hours a day and consuming all calories inside an eight-hour span. Women are recommended to begin with 14-hour fasting and gradually increasing to 16 hours.

Whatever option you select, it is critical to eat well during non-fasting hours. If you consume many fatty, calorie-dense meals during your non-fasting hours, you will not get the same weight reduction and health benefits. In the end, the right solution is to be tolerated and maintained for the long run and without a detrimental effect on your wellbeing.

5.1. Schedule for Intermittent Fasting for Beginners

We always suggest beginning with the most common and beginner-friendly form, Intermittent Fasting 16/8; We suggest transitioning into Intermittent Fasting by beginning with 12 hours of fasting and 12 hours of eating, incorporating one fasting hour per day before you hit the targeted 16/8 schedule.

5.2. What Do You Eat During Intermittent Fasting?

A common myth is that you can eat whatever you want when doing Intermittent Fasting, like sugary desserts, fast food, and heavily refined foods. It is important to stick to nutritious meals if you want to lose weight, increase efficiency, or even get healthier. It means consuming whole foods and ignoring the normal suspects, including empty carbohydrates, processed foods, sugars, and so on.

It is entirely up to you the diet you follow if it is well-balanced and suits your lifestyle. Keto Diet was a perfect addition to Intermittent Fasting for many, enabling them to burn more fat.

5.3. What Do You Drink During Intermittent Fasting?

To reap all the health benefits of Intermittent Fasting, such as weight loss, higher metabolic rate, reduced blood sugar levels, immune system improvement. So on, it would help if you refrained from eating any caloric food. On the other hand, noncaloric drinks do not break your fast and encourage you to reap all the benefits of fasting. It is because noncaloric drinks do not induce insulin release and, as a result, do not mess with fat burning and autophagy (cellular cleanup). This will contain the following:

- Water
- Sparkling Water
- Mineral Water
- Black Coffee
- Plain Tea

5.4. Advice from Experts on Intermittent Fasting

It is important to have a regular eating schedule. Consistency with the schedule has been shown to yield improved outcomes, as we mentioned in our interview with Intermittent Fasting specialist Dr. Jason Fung's associate and clinical scholar Megan J. Ramos. Here are few pointers to make your life easier:

Begin with an overhauled plan. Begin with a manageable schedule and gradually increase the pace and duration. There is no reason to jump right in! Develop your tolerance to eating in a smaller time window per day, then progress to the full schedule when you are ready.

Maintain hydration. During your fasting time, stay hydrated with "noncaloric fluids." Herbal teas, water, and calorie-free flavored drinks are examples of such beverages.

Eat steadily and regularly during feeding time. Experts suggest aiming to eat every 3 hours during the 8-hour timeframe to "get all your calories." Mind that IF can be harmful if you do not consume the required number of calories a day.

Get a healthy, nutritious plan. Although it may be tempting to indulge in your favorite comfort foods and snacks until your fasting time is over, strictly adhere to a balanced diet rich in proteins, vegetables, and fruits.

Make your menus ahead of time. If your life is very hectic, set aside some time on the weekend or a couple of times a week to plan some meals ahead of time. It will save you time and assist you in maintaining a healthy diet.

Adding 2-3 tablespoons of fat to your evening meal. To keep blood glucose levels stable overnight, a resident dietitian for Sovereign Labs advises having a healthy, good fat like avocado olive oil or coconut butter in the last meal of the day.

If you have difficulty sleeping, IF may not be for you. If you do not sleep through the night, do not try this strategy, says an IF specialist. Priority should be given to sleep.

Chapter 6.

INTERMITTENT FASTING FOOD LIST

Consuming food while intermittent fasting is more about maintaining a healthier lifestyle than it is about quickly losing weight. As a result, it is important to select nutrient-rich foods, such as fruits, vegetables, lean proteins, and good fats.

The list of intermittent fasting foods should include the following:

6.1. Hydration

The National Academies of Sciences & Medicine recommends approximately.

- 3.7 liters (15.5 cups) of fluid a day for men.

- 2.7 liters (11.5 cups) of fluid a day for ladies

Liquids include both pure water and beverages and foods containing water. Maintaining enough hydration is critical for your health during intermittent fasting. Dehydration can manifest itself in the form of headaches, intense fatigue, and dizziness. And if you are still experiencing some of these fasting side effects, dehydration will exacerbate or even trigger them. The following foods are included on the intermittent fasting food list for hydration:

- Water

- Sparkling or Mineral Water

- Tea or Black Coffee

- Plain Yogurt

- Strawberries

- Watermelon

- Peaches

- Oranges

- Skim Milk

- Tomatoes

- Lettuce

- Celery

Importantly, drinking lots of water will aid in weight loss as well. According to a 2016 analysis article, adequate hydration will aid in weight loss by:

- Enhance fat burning.

- Minimizing appetite or intake of food

Foods to Avoid When Intermittent Fasting

- Processed Meat

- Trans-Fat

- Refined Grain

- Processed Foods

- Alcoholic Beverages

- Sugar-Sweetened Beverages

- Candy Bars

6.2. Fats

According to the Dietary Guidelines, 2015 - 2020 for Americans, which advocate replacing saturated fat with unsaturated fat, a person's maximum caloric intake should be 20% to 35% of total daily calories. Notably, saturated fat does not exceed 10% of daily calories.

Fats may be beneficial, harmful, or anywhere in between, based on the type of Vegetable oils, such as increasing inflammation, lowering "good" cholesterol levels, and raising "bad" cholesterol levels. They are present in baked and fried foods.

Saturated fats have been linked to an increased risk of heart disease. However, expert views on this subject vary. It is prudent to consume them in moderation. Saturated fats are abundant in whole milk, red meat, baked goods, and coconut oil. Monounsaturated and polyunsaturated fats are considered healthy fats. Such fats have been shown to decrease the risk of heart failure, lower blood pressure, and lower fat levels in the blood. These fats are found in olive oil, peanut oil, canola oil, safflower oil, sunflower oil, and soybean oils.

The following foods are included on the IF fats list:

- Nuts

- Whole Eggs

- Dark Chocolate

- Full Fat Yogurt

- Chia Seeds

- Avocados

- Fatty Fish

- Cheese

- Olive Oil (Extra Virgin)

6.3. Protein

The daily recommended protein allowance (D.R.I.) is the level required for adults is 0.8 g of protein per kg of your weight. Your specifications can differ according to your fitness objectives and level of exercise.

Protein aids in weight loss by reducing energy intake, speeding up metabolism, and increasing satiety. Additionally, when paired with strength exercise, enhanced protein consumption aids in muscle development. Muscle burns more calories than fat, so possessing more muscle naturally raises the metabolism. According to a recent report, having more muscles in your legs can help prevent the development of belly fat in healthy men.

Protein-rich foods on the IF food list include the following:

- Poultry and Fish

- Eggs

- Seafood

- Dairy Products (e.g., milk, yogurt, and cheese)

- Nuts and Seeds.

- Legumes & Beans

- Soy

- Whole Grains

6.4. Carbs

According to the American Dietetic Association, carbohydrates can account for 45 to 65 percent of daily calories (carbs). Carbohydrates are the body's primary source of energy. Fat and protein are the remaining two. Carbohydrates come in a variety of kinds; sugar, fiber, and starch are the most notable.

Carbohydrates often get a poor reputation for contributing to weight gain. Carbohydrates, however, are not necessarily made equal and are not simply fattening. Whether or not you gain weight is dependent on the form and amount of carbohydrates you consume.

Pick foods that are low in sugar but rich in fiber and starch. According to a 2015 report, eating 30g of fiber daily will help you lose weight, enhance your glucose levels, and reduce blood pressure. Consuming 30g of fiber a day is not difficult. They can be obtained by consuming a plain egg sandwich, Mediterranean barley with chickpeas, apple with peanut butter, or chicken and black pea enchiladas.

The following foods are included on the IF carbohydrate list:

- Quinoa

- Oats

- Brown Rice

- Apples

- Banana

- Berries

- Mangoes

- Pears

- Kidneys Beans

- Sweet Potatoes

- Beetroots

- Broccoli

- Avocados

- Brussels Sprouts

- Carrots

- Chickpeas

- Chia Seed

- Nuts

6.5. A Healthy Gut

Recent studies prove that your overall wellbeing depends on your digestive system's power. Your gut contains billions of bacteria collectively referred to as the microbiota. These bacteria affect the health of your gut, metabolism, and mental wellbeing. Additionally, they can play a critical role in a variety of chronic conditions. As a precaution, you must take care of these tiny bugs in the gut, even more so if you are fasting intermittently.

The following foods are included on the intermittent fasting food page for a balanced gut:

- All Vegetables

- Tempeh

- Fermented Vegetables

- Kefir

- Sauerkraut

- Kimchi

- Miso

- Kombucha

Along with maintaining a balanced stomach, these foods can aid in weight loss by

- Reducing fat absorption from the stomach

- Increasing the amount of fat excreted in the stools.

- Consumption of food is being reduced.

Chapter 7.

MEAL SCHEDULING FOR INTERMITTENT FASTING

Although the concept of fasting can be intimidating, particularly if you have never done this before, intermittent fasting can be much simpler than certain other methods of eating plans.

When you begin your intermittent fasting phase, you will most soon recognize that you feel fuller for longer periods of time and that you can make the meals simpler and easy for you to eat. There are several ways to fast, so we have divided each of the strategies below into beginner, moderate, and advanced, providing a standard meal plan with each.

The combined effect of the nutrients will provide you with the fuel you require to reap the effectiveness of your fasting process. Consider making an account for any personal food intolerances or allergies, and adjust your diet according to your specific health situation,

Try to Learn: Mind that intermittent fasting does not always imply calorie restriction, so eat per your caloric requirements.

Cure with Food: Make educated food decisions to treat autoimmune disease, inflammation, and other chronic conditions.

7.1. A Beginner's Intermittent Fasting Meal Strategy

If you are new to fasting, the perfect way to get into the flow is to eat between 8 a.m. and 6 p.m. This schedule encourages you to eat all three meals and some snacks while still fasting for 14 hours in a 24-hour span.

Breakfast 8 a.m. - green smoothie.

After the 14hr fast, start your day with a smoothie as it will be easier to digest. Go for a green smoothie to avoid getting on a blood-sugar roller coaster with a high-sugar banana smoothie. Be sure to have plenty of good fats to fill you up till lunch!

How to prepare:

- One avocado

- One cup of coconut milk

- A small handful of blueberries

- One cup of greens (kale, spinach, or chard)

- One teaspoon chia seed

Procedure:

1. Combine all ingredients in a blender, mix, and serve!

Lunch: Noon, Grass-Fed Burgers

Grass-fed liver burgers are incredibly simple to prepare for the whole week. Enjoy it over a bed of fiber-rich greens with a basic homemade sauce for a nutritious meal full of B vitamins.

How to prepare:

- Half pound of grass-fed field beef

- Half pound of grass-fed beef liver

- Half tsp cumin powder

- Half tsp garlic powder

- Sea salt & pepper to taste

- Cooking oil

Procedure:

1. Combine all ingredients in a mixing bowl and shape into preferred size patties.

2. In a pan, heat Cooking oil over med-high heat

3. Cook the burgers in skillet until done per taste.

4. Keep in a container to use within four days.

Snack: 2:30 p.m. Fat Bombs "Cinnamon Roll."

Fat bombs will indulge your sugar craving while providing sufficient healthy fats to keep you going till dinner, and they taste particularly good because they taste like cinnamon rolls.

How to prepare:

- Half a cup of coconut cream

- One teaspoon ground cinnamon

- One tablespoon coconut oil

- Two tbsp almond butter

Procedure:

1. Combine the coconut cream and half a teaspoon of cinnamon in a mixing bowl.

2. Line an 8x8-inch baking pan (square) with butter paper and layer the cinnamon mixture and coconut cream evenly on the bottom.

3. Combine the remaining half teaspoon of cinnamon, almond butter, and coconut oil in a mixing bowl. Layer it over the pan's first layer.

4. Chill for 10 minutes before cutting into bars or squares.

Dinner: 5:30 p.m. salmon and vegetables.

Salmon is rich in omega-3 fatty fats, while dark green vegetables, including broccoli and kale, are full of antioxidants. Salmon is one of my personal favorites because of its flavor and nutrient abundance, but you can use any wild-caught seafood you choose. Serve with your favorite roasted veggies in coconut oil for a simple and convenient superfood dinner.

How to prepare:

- One pound of salmon or any type of seafood

- Two tbsp. of fresh lemon juice

- Two tbsp. pure ghee

- Four cloves of garlic, finely minced

Procedure:

1. Heat the oven to 400°F.

2. Combine the lemon juice, garlic, and ghee, in a mixing bowl.

3. Placing the salmon in a foil, drizzle with the lemon-ghee mixture.

4. Fold the salmon in the foil and set it on a baking tray.

5. Bake for about 15 minutes, or till the salmon is cooked thoroughly.

6. If the oven is large enough, roast your vegetables on a separate baking tray alongside the salmon.

7.2. An Intermediate's Intermittent Fasting Meal Strategy

This strategy requires you to eat only between the hours of 12 p.m. and 6 p.m. for a total of 18 hours of fasting over a 24-hour span.

This plan can be put into action During the workweek. Skip breakfast and start your day with a few cups of herbal tea.

If you do not drink tea, it is important that you remain hydrated. Drink plenty of water while you are at it. You may also drink herbal tea (most experts believe that coffee and tea do not break the fast). Tea catechins have been shown to increase the benefits of fasting by decreasing the appetite hormone ghrelin, allowing you to fast before lunch without feeling deprived.

Since you have added four hours to your fasting time, ensure your first lunch (at noon) contains sufficiently good fats. The burger will fit great with the 8-to-6-window plan, and you can add more fats with your sauce or top with avocado!

Seeds and nuts are high-fat treats that can be consumed at 2:30 p.m. Soaking these ahead of time will help neutralize naturally occurring enzymes such as phytates, which can lead to digestive issues.

Dinner will be at 5:30 p.m., and, as with the 8-to-6-window menu, a dinner of wild-caught salmon or another clean source of protein with vegetables is a perfect choice.

Lunch: 12 p.m., Grass-fed burger with avocado (first meal)

Snack: 2:30 p.m. Seeds and nuts

Dinner: 5:30 p.m. Salmon and vegetables

7.3. An Advanced Intermittent Fasting Meal Strategy: The Modified 2-Day Meal Plan
Eating clean for five days a week in this program (you can pick whatever days you want). Limit your calories to no more than 700 a day on the other two days. Calorie restriction provides much of the same advantages as a full-day fast.

On non-fasting days, make sure you are consuming enough good fats, lean foods, veggies, and fruits, and you should plan your meals as they works better for you.

On controlled days, you can eat smaller meals or snacks during the day, or you can eat a moderate-sized lunch and dinner and short throughout the morning and after dinner. Focus on good fats, clean proteins, and produce once more. Apps could assist you with logging your diet and keeping track of your calorie consumption so that you do not exceed 700.

7.4. A Super Advanced Intermittent Fasting Meal Strategy: 5-2 Meal Plan.

Under this schedule, you can eat normal and healthy five days a week and for two nonconsecutive days do not eat anything. For, e.g., fast on Mondays and Thursdays but eat healthy meals the rest of the week. These five days' food will be like the rest of the fasting plans, with good fats, clean meat products, vegetables, and some fruit.

Remember that this schedule is not for beginners, and you should always consult with your doctor before beginning any fasting regimen, particularly if you are taking medicine or have a medical condition. It is advised that coffee drinkers continue to drink their morning coffee and that anyone who participates in an advanced fast remains well hydrated.

Monday: Fasting

Tuesday: Consume healthier lean meats, fats, veggies, and fruit.

Wednesday: Consume lean meats, good fats, veggies, and fruit.

Thursday: Fasting

Friday: Consume lean meats, balanced fats, veggies, and berries.

Saturday: Consume lean meats, balanced fats, veggies, and fruit.

7.5. Expert-Level Intermittent Fasting Meal Strategy: Alternate-Day Fasting.

About its complexity, this strategy is very straightforward. You should not eat every other day. Eat clean meat sources, good fats, vegetables, and a little fruit every single day, and then on fasting days, drink herbal tea, water, and moderate quantities of black tea or coffee.

Monday: Consume lean meats, good fats, veggies and fruit.

Tuesday: Fasting.

Wednesday: Consume lean meats, good fats, veggies and fruit.

Thursday: Fasting.

Friday: Consume lean meats, good fats, veggies and fruit.

Saturday: Fasting.

Sunday: Consume lean meats, good fats, veggies and fruit.

With this knowledge, you should be able to prepare your meals before beginning an intermittent fasting plan. And, while it may be difficult at first, but when you get into the rhythm of fasting, it will become second nature and blend into your days easily. However, always begin slowly and eventually progress to more progressed plans.

It is also significant to mention that intermittent fasting will not work for you on certain days. Pay attention to your body—it is fine if you need to feed outside your usual window. Simply restart when you feel better.

Chapter 8.

BRING IT ON!

After all the information and knowledge bombarded at you, you must be eager to get going with your fast. But Along with understanding your fitness priorities, take the following precautions before getting into IF:

Consult your primary care physician. A health practitioner will ascertain whether this eating style is helpful to the body. "If you have any concerns about what is best for you, it is important to speak with healthcare professionals," an IF expert advises. "Everyone is unique, and your physician may have recommendations for what you should do and not do in light of your unique circumstances."

Select the appropriate kind of IF for you. If you always socialize late at night, for example, 5:2 is likely to be a better match than 16:8. If you wish to give 16:8 a chance, experts advise that you begin slowly. "I suggest beginning slowly and gradually starting with a 12-hr fast and a 12-hr eating window, then progressing to a 14-hr fast and a 10-hr eating window, and finally to get to 16:8," they say. Additionally, the importance of maintaining a flexible eating and fasting window is much emphasized. "Some people like to eat at noon and stop at 8 p.m. Determine what is best for you.

Ensure proper hydration. The 2019 Nutrient report recommends consuming lots of water each day to prevent dehydration and improve the replacement of the fluids you would get from food consumption.

Restricted Physical activity. Moreover, limiting your movements during your fasting windows till you know how the body will respond recommend some IF experts.

8.1. 3 Essential Suggestions

1. There are several fasting techniques.

Certain individuals fast for 9 hours, some for 20 hours, or even longer. Others drastically reduce their calorie intake over a specified number of days per week or per month.

The famous "5:2" schedule requires two days of weekly caloric restriction. On fasting days, you consume two meals (approximately 500 calories in total). On days when you are not fasting, you maintain a balanced diet but do not limit calories.

2. Importance of meal planning.

Experts say you must get enough nutrients before you start a fast and after.

Healthy meals to consume prior to a fast include the following:

- Fruits and veggies (these will help with hydration).

- Lean protein-rich foods, such as fish or chicken.

- Yogurt with reduced fat.

- High-sodium foods should be avoided as they can induce bloating, like pizza and canned soup.

3. Then break the fast gradually.

When you finish fasting, do not immediately begin eating anything in sight.

Otherwise, you will shock the system; it is better to begin with dried fruit or a few dates. After that, take a break and begin with fruit or other light foods.

You have likely even participated in several periodic fasts in your life.

If you had late dinner, then slept late, and then skipped lunch the next day, you may have now fasted for 16+ hours. Some individuals feed in this manner unconsciously. They may not have an appetite in the morning.

Most people regard the 16/8 approach to be the most straightforward and sustainable method of intermittent fasting; you may want to give it a try first. When you feel comfortable and healthy while fasting, you can progress to more extreme fasts such as 24-hr fasts a few times a week (Eat-Stop-Eat) or consuming 500–600 calories a few days a week (5:2 diet).

8.2. How to Begin

Getting started is simplistic. Indeed, odds are you have already participated in several sporadic fasts. Many people eat this way instinctively, avoiding breakfast and dinner.

The simplest way to begin is to choose one of the intermittent fasting strategies mentioned above and give it a try. However, you are not required to adhere to a formal schedule. Alternatively, it would help if you fasted anytime it is convenient for you. Skipping meals on occasion when you are not hungry or lack time to prepare them can work for most people. There is no need to adhere to a formal intermittent fasting regimen in order to reap some of the advantages of IF.

Experiment with various ways before you discover one that appeals to you and suits your timetable. At the end of the day, it makes no difference which fasting method you select. The critical factor is to determine which approach fits well for you and your lifestyle.

8.3. Intermittent Fasting Side Effects & Their Cures

It is a normal phenomenon – you make lifestyle changes and wind up feeling weaker than you did already. Fasting on an intermittent basis is no different. Although it is not necessarily the case, intermittent fasting adverse effects do occur on occasion. Especially within the first few weeks as your body adjusts to the changes.

As you notice the consequences of modifying your diet, it is important to understand that you can mitigate these side effects in advance. Never be afraid. When you launch a new lifestyle or switch back to one after a break, you can overcome your body's initial response.

Intermittent fasting can be accomplished in various ways, including OMAD or feeding within a defined time window. Based on the form of fasting you chose, the initial side effects will range from mild to serious. However, most side effects will subside within the first week. None can last more than a few weeks. Your body will simply adapt with time.

Among the adverse effects are the following:

- Headaches

- Flu-like Symptoms

- Hair Loss

- Brain fog

- Overeating

- Sleep Disturbance

- Bowel Issues

- Negative Medication Interactions

All these adverse effects will be discussed in-depth further down.

The Most Common Adverse Effects of Intermittent Fasting

Headaches

Headaches are one of the most frequent side effects of intermittent fasting within the first week. Headaches also arise as the body responds to a shift in dietary patterns. If your body is dehydrated, it will warn you. You begin to experience a dry throat or a heaviness in your mouth. Water deficiency is a significant side effect of dehydration. It cannot be emphasized enough how important it is to closely track your water consumption during the initial intermittent fasting period. Another possibility for a headache is that you are used to consuming tea or some other caffeinated beverage and decreasing caffeine consumption through fasting.

Symptoms of Flu

Have you awoken today feeling a little under the weather? Rather than worrying about contracting the plague, consider when the symptoms began. Did they begin shortly after you began fasting? As in most diets, you might undergo a time during which you feel as though you are heading towards the flu. It is indicated by fasting pains, fatigue, and an overall feeling of weariness. You can also have nausea associated with intermittent fasting.

Avoid reaching for the closest flu drug to assist with alleviating these effects. Hydration is the true cure. Ensure that you consume sufficient water with electrolytes to alleviate these effects. There are several guidelines on the quantity of fluid consumption, but the best approach is to decide the appropriate amount depending on how you honestly feel. As a rule, drink approximately 2 liters of water or 8 glasses of 8 oz water a day.

That is because when you start intermittent fasting, the body quickly removes extra water. Consequently, essential electrolytes are lost, and you become dehydrated. Therefore, you must immediately replace these to prevent becoming ill.

Hair Loss

The most worrying side effect of IF is hair loss. However, you do not need to be concerned about it excessively. When you practice intermittent fasting, you are likely to experience some hair loss. You ingest fewer calories when fasting than you would usually. As a result, you are more likely to consume less food. Your body responds to calorie restriction in a variety of ways, one of which is hair loss.

Although it may seem as though you are balding, but this is not the case. Hair loss is normal at first and can resolve on its own. When it does not, begin monitoring your food intake to ensure you get the proper amount of nutrients and calories. You must always ensure that you have enough nutrients to keep the body in order.

Brain Fog

The most noticeable and frequent side effect of attempting a new diet is brain fog. You can experience forgetfulness, fatigue, or an inability to focus as you did before. You can also experience restlessness as a result of brain fog. Although it is uncomfortable, brain fog is not a sign of poor health.

When you start to fast intermittently, brain fog quickly sets in. When you walk into the kitchen and have no idea why you went there, you know the fog has set in. It is infuriating when your head is foggy, but there are things you can do to help alleviate it. The most effective approach to combat brain fog is to take regular breaks when doing challenging activities. Every hour or so, take a short stroll. Another way to combat the fogginess is to ensure that you get enough sleep. And do not try to eliminate the fogginess by infusing yourself with a steady supply of caffeine. It would not be beneficial in the long run.

Overeating

Fasting does one thing more than anything else: it stimulates appetite. When your eating window approaches, you might l find yourself tempted to consume both the food and the plate. It is not rare, to begin with, ravenous hunger. You do not want to overindulge during your window, as this would undermine your efforts. As a rule, ensure that you consume lots of water while feeding. Consume mindfully; your brain takes up to 20 minutes to acknowledge that you are full; allow your brain to keep pace with your fork.

Drink Tea. A calorie-free beverage will fool your mind into believing you are drinking something substantial. Tea is an outstanding alternative because it keeps you satiated and is permitted in the fasting window.

Bowel Disorders

While discussing bowel movements may seem poopy, you should know that intermittent fasting may cause constipation or even fasting diarrhea. Inability to go to the toilet or excessive urination is one of the most unpleasant side effects. This happens as a result of the body depleting nutrients or not consuming enough water.

There are numerous natural methods to assist with the progression of events (in the intestines!). One effective method is to increase water intake. Another solution is to consume more fiber during the feeding window. Ascertain that the diet is well-balanced to avoid deficiency in vital nutrients. Having difficulty getting things going, you should consider altering your diet. In addition to water, you can consume natural laxatives such as prunes, prune juice, cranberry juice, and figs. Ensure that you are having enough amount of dietary fiber.

Disturbance in Sleep

There has been much debate about sleep and intermittent fasting. Although some claim that fasting helps them sleep better, a few reports experiencing sleep disturbances due to fasting. Among the most obvious explanations may be because you are starving. Sleeping is difficult when you are hungry.

Another explanation you might be having trouble sleeping is because you are worried about food. Food dreams, food imaginations, and food desires. Though you may have insomnia for a few hours, it will subside, and you may find you are sleeping better than ever.

Negative Medication Interactions

You must ensure that your taking medications will not have an adverse effect while you are fasting. Consult your physician first. Although fasting has many advantages, it can be riskier when taking medications. Some health problems can deteriorate as a result of dietary restrictions and feeding at specific hours. Individuals with diabetes should exercise caution when fasting. Such disorders are those associated with heart disease or hypertension.

Give It A Chance

Never be afraid. - When you begin a new plan, you must anticipate that it will take some time for your body to adjust. As in any lifestyle modifications, these effects can subside within a

week or two if you remain stable. Just do not surrender if you are having trouble getting the full benefits of intermittent fasting's detrimental effects will wear off quickly, and you will reap some outstanding benefits.

And once adverse effects of intermittent fasting subside, you will benefit tremendously. You will soon notice that you can think more clearly, have more stamina, and begin losing weight. After you have gotten through the difficult part, you may ask why you did not start earlier.

Chapter 9.

INTERMITTENT FASTING & PHYSICAL ACTIVITY

If you believe IF an aspect is you want to add to your lifestyle, the challenge is to include some sort of physical activity comfortably when doing so. After all, the food we consume becomes the body's fuel when we exercise. Intermittent fasting involves going long periods without consuming some food or drink, let alone the carbohydrates or protein we usually equate with performance eating.

How to exercise while fasting intermittently:

9.1. Pay Attention to The Body

Begin by maintaining cardio exercises at an aerobic pace when fasting, ensuring that you can always converse. Although the performance can probably suffer, recent research indicates that if players retain their overall calorie and nutritional consumption and their normal quality of sleep, they are unlikely to experience any detrimental effects on performance. Therefore, if you feel as though you are testing the limits of your body, do not be afraid to pause.

It is not to say that something is wrong; it could mean that you need to continue training and determining the level of stress you can handle in the coming weeks.

9.2. Perform High-Intensity Exercises After Eating

If you are approaching a difficult or intensive training block, now may not be the best time to begin fasting. Certain sessions may be completed while fasting; however, bear in mind that they can feel more difficult than normal. Consider timing your strenuous exercises after meals to ensure that you have enough resources to fuel your body.

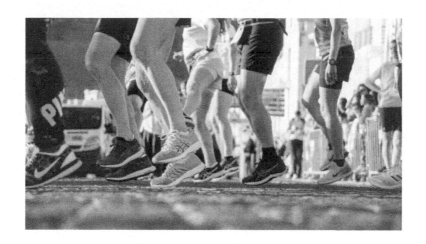

Of course, healing is critical because if you do a difficult session while fasting and maintain the fast, you will become deficient in essential nutrients for recoveries, such as carbohydrates and protein. It reduces the benefit of exercise and makes you more susceptible to sickness and injury. Again, carefully schedule the tougher or more demanding exercises to allow for enough rehabilitation and exercise gains.

9.3. Hydrate Your Body

Hydration is always essential, but it is more needed when exercising and fasting. We are aware that electrolytes are depleted by sweat and that they must be replenished. Any fast lasting longer than 12 hours raises the risk of electrolyte depletion. There are now fewer electrolytes absorbed from food and because low insulin levels allow the kidney to excrete more electrolytes than normal.

Obviously just drinking water is insufficient; it is critical to replenish the electrolytes with a sugar-free formula such as Bindilyte to ensure the body receives the potassium, sodium, calcium and magnesium, it needs daily.

Although in intermittent fasting, the optimal time to exercise is normally immediately upon awakening or shortly afterward to maintain the body's normal circadian rhythm. Exercising (or eating) near bedtime has been shown to disrupt R.E.M. stages and deep sleep, so it is best to reserve exercise for the next day.

In an idealistic situation, you would avoid eating immediately after an exercise for the same reason you would avoid exercising in a fasted state: hormone optimization. [[Even waiting two to three hours following a workout before eating promotes an increase in growth hormone, which makes you become a fat burner and replaces the energy you used during the workout (sugar). A hormone change happens as a result of an adjustment to the pressure caused by a high-intensity exercise. If your routine only allows for a workout at lunchtime, you can exercise during your time available and then reap the hormonal benefits by abstaining from food for two to three hours after your workout.

9.4. Cardiovascular Exercise & Intermittent Fasting

The hormonal gains of fasted exercise are due to the liver glycogen reserves and reduced muscle that develops during fasting. However, exercise is suitable for intermittent fasting; the success will be determined by how fat-enhanced your body is (i.e., does it burn burning fat for fuel). If you are new to fasting and exercising, your results will suffer slightly; it may take around six months for certain athletes to complete this new energy e source transition. For instance, if you are a competitive swimmer whose primary focus is race efficiency, do not turn to fasted training just a few weeks before a contest.

If you like doing cardio while fasting, do not prolong the fast post-workout rather, choose to refill afterward.

9.5. Sprint Training & Intermittent Fasting

HIIT, high-intensity interval training or sprint training consists of 15–30-minute periods of intense physical exercise followed by rest. Sprint training time is Not only efficient, but research indicates that it offers health benefits not achievable from aerobic activity alone, such as a substantial increase in HGH (human growth hormone). Sprint exercise has many advantages, including enhanced endurance, brainpower and muscle, increased growth hormone, improved brain activity, improved body structure, decreased depression, and increased testosterone levels. Many of these advantages are enhanced when sprint running is combined with intermittent fasting. Sprint training is the optimal exercise strategy to integrate with your fasted state, and you should continue fasting for two to three hours after a workout to maximize the benefits.

9.6. Weight-lifting and Intermittent Fasting

Lifting weights while fasting is also appropriate, but you must keep in mind the role of glucose in muscle recovery after strenuous weight-lifting activity, especially while fasting. When you exercise while fasting, the glycogen reserves are exhausted. If your day's exercise includes heavy lifting, you can do it while fasting, but you should consider eating a nutritious meal immediately after that.

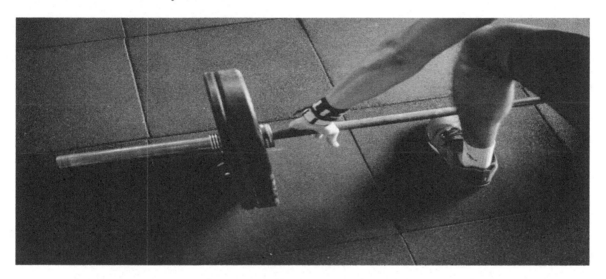

Unlike a burst workout session, heavy lifting places the body under such tension that it requires an urgent refeed. As with cardio, lifting weights while fasting can temporarily reduce your strength as your body adjusts to being a "fat burner." As a result, you may want to schedule weight-lifting workouts after meals (in this case, you can break your fast after two to three hours of workout) and introduce fasted exercise on days where you do burst-style training.

Chapter 10.

REMAINING FIT AND WELL AFTER 50

For women, reaching the age of 50 is a significant achievement. Society informs you that you are at a crossroads. Your physical appearance emphasizes the argument. Any woman over the age of 50 is aware of it. Connect with your mind and body – they will take you wherever you want to go. These pointers will get you moving.

"Children are off to university, and parents are elderly. There may be marital difficulties or employment difficulties. It is unquestionably a difficult moment, "Jennifer Zreloff, MD, is an internist for Emory University School of Medicine's executive wellness program. "Additionally, you discover that you cannot manipulate your body as often as you did when you were young. Your body is just not as powerful as it once was. This is a moment for women to take a hard look at their lifestyle choices and make some adjustments."

According to a retirement lifestyle expert in Norwalk, Conn, it is also a moment of self-reflection for many women over 50. "You begin to consider your life's purpose, about discovering what brings you joy and content. You might be ready for a change, for work that you enjoy."

Enhancing the Body and Mind

To keep your body and mind in peak condition, here is your to-do list:

Adopt a positive attitude. Pause and consider what you expect from life. Discover your objective and purpose. Then share that joy with others.

Exercise regularly, like walking or aerobics. It strengthens the bones. Additionally, it lowers the risk of developing heart failure. Heart disease is the leading cause of death in women.

Allocate reflective time each morning. Consider meditating, praying, and visualizing the day. Read something inspiring. Concentrate on self-renewal.

Sleep well. Perhaps you got by with four hours of sleep a night in your 40's, but your body cannot handle the deprivation as you age.

Have an annual physical examination. Your cholesterol, blood pressure, thyroid levels and glucose should all be tested. Additionally, discuss with your psychiatrist some signs of depression, which are normal in women over 50. These include constant or pessimism, depression, feelings of hopelessness, worthlessness, concentration difficulties, insomnia and anxiety.

Secure yourself against cancer. Mammograms should be performed on an annual basis. Colon screening is recommended starting at the age of 50. If you are sexually active, Pap smears should be repeated after one or three years.

Λ bone density scan can be used to determine the density of the bones. Consult your physician on vitamin d, and Calcium Regular calcium intake should be at least 1,200 milligrams.

Recommended

Introduce yourself to yoga. Yoga is an excellent stretching technique that also improves endurance. Flexibility improves equilibrium and prevents falls and fractures.

Get some fun. Bungee jumping, rock climbing, backpacking, hiking, and dancing are all great ways to spend your time. Act as if you are feeling it, and you can feel more youthful.

Drink sensibly. One alcoholic drink a night is appropriate for all women, not just those over 50.

Consume vibrant products. Women over the age of 50 need to consume a variety of vegetables and fruits. Additionally, consume more fatty fish (such as salmon) to get omega-3, heart-healthy fatty acids. Develop an appreciation for lentils, whole grains, and skinless lean protein sources. Let yourself occasional indulgences in desserts. When choosing oils, err on the side of caution and go for high-quality varieties such as extra-virgin olive oil.

Locate an outlet for your creativity. It aids in the prevention of depression — and depression impairs memory. Having an artistic outlet aids in brain stimulation. Create an amazing garden. Consider taking up painting. Participating in creative endeavors challenges the imagination more than reading and more than watching television.

Convert your house into an oasis. Eliminate accumulated clutter. Enhance your life with wonderful songs, books, and people you care about. When required, withdraw and recharge.

Associating with those who are optimistic is beneficial. They would not squander your precious resources on grievances. They will assist you in pursuing the best aspects of life. With women over 50, the quest can take on any shape and take them anywhere. Make the most of your life right now.

Chapter 11.

INTERMITTENT FASTING MYTHS

Men and women of all ages have gotten on board this diet and wellness movement in order to assist them in losing weight and improving their health. Before you follow in the footsteps of supposed followers, you should be clear about how this kind of "diet" really means.

According to the author of the health-focused book, Dr. Zembroski, while fasting has been beneficial for the mind and body, there are certain risks associated with it. "Those who fast often consume high-fat, high-calorie foods under the mistaken belief that fasting allows them to consume whatever they want," he said. "Whenever the body is deprived of food, there is a physiological urge to overeat leading to the activation of appetite hormones such as leptin and ghrelin, as well as activation of the brain's hunger center. This would result in people overeating following their fast."

To assist you on your trip, here are ten misconceptions about intermittent fasting that have been debunked.

Myth: When you break your fast, you can eat as much as you would like.

You can continue to consume meals of normal size.

Intermittent fasting — like any other diet — is just the beginning of the journey toward a healthy lifestyle. Sadly, many assume that after their fast is over, they will resume disordered eating.

And, according to experts, doing so would essentially negate all the efforts.

The trick to success with I.F. is to eat normally after your fast. If you fast all day until dinner and only consume a dinner the size of breakfast/lunch/dinner, all at once, you have effectively negated the time spent fasting."

Myth: Fasting causes the metabolism to slow down.

You need not be calorie-limited.

If you are afraid or excited at the prospect of slowing your metabolism by intermittent fasting, experts assert that this is a misconception, and they are here to refute it.

"The aim of intermittent fasting is not to limit calories; it is to restrict the period during which calories are eaten," they explained. "Delaying your first meal by a few hours would have little effect on your metabolic rate. Changes in metabolic function arise due to undereating — and does not occur on an intermittent fasting diet."

Myth: Intermittent fasting is effective since the body does not digest food throughout the night.

Rest assured that even if you feed at 3 a.m., the body will process it.

One of the most pervasive myths about fasting is the way it functions. As it is often believed that digestion ceases after a certain period, this is not the case.

The body can digest food regardless of the time. It is a matter of giving the body enough time (whether researchers agree on 10-12-16 hours is an open question) to concentrate on other physiological processes such as cellular repair and autophagy rather than diverting resources to digestion. Rest easy knowing that even if you feed at 3 a.m., the body will process it.

Myth: Fasting is more effective for weight loss than snacking.

It is dependent on the snack's calorie content.

When dieting, it is sometimes suggested that you should snack between meals. However, one of the most prevalent misconceptions about intermittent fasting leads those who attempt it to believe that it can be used in place of balanced snacking.

Ultimately, weight loss is a feature of maintaining a steady calorie deficit. It makes no difference if such calories are eaten during the day or in a four to eight-hour cycle. Do what is right for your lifestyle and body in order to achieve the goals set."

Myth: All intermittent fasting is identical and produces identical outcomes.

Each person's body will react differently to fasting.

Contrary to popular opinion, there are many ways of intermittent fasting. Intermittent fasting does not have an "official" definition. Additionally, there are several varieties.

Many I.F. guidelines require complete fasting every single day, while others require a certain number of calories or time-restricted feeding within a six, eight, or ten-hour span per day.

Myth: It is difficult to exercise when fasting.

It is possible to exercise while fasting.

According to a certified fitness nutrition expert and an A.C.E. certified personal trainer, exercising while fasting is potentially beneficial.

In fact, the optimal time to exercise is first thing in the morning on an empty stomach, he said. This way, you will be burning fat already deposited on your body rather than the calories from your recent meal. Consume breakfast after your exercise to refuel your body.

Myth: Fasting for losing weight is more effective than other methods of weight loss.

Calorie restriction in any form can result in weight loss.

If you believe that intermittent fasting is the safest method for weight loss, you may want to reconsider. At its most fundamental level, intermittent fasting is a type of caloric restriction. Intermittent fasting is not more effective than other ways and methods of weight loss.

Myth: You can lose weight regardless of what you do.

Weight reduction is not a sure thing.

Contrary to common opinion, extended fasting — or, more broadly, fasting — would not necessarily result in weight loss. It is a general misunderstanding about this form of dieting.

It makes no difference how long the fasting is; if you break it with burgers, pizza, and candy, the results will be slim to zero. I.F. operates in conjunction with a balanced diet. Each fasting day cannot be regarded as a cheat day if the diet is to be effective.

Myth: A large breakfast is needed since it is regarded as an essential meal of the day.

Consume foods that are beneficial to the health.

Though it is commonly believed that you can consume enough breakfast to sustain your day, but this is not always the case. Breakfast is a significant part of American culture, a hearty, full breakfast. Of course, cereal makers want you to believe that, but the truth is that you must listen to your body and have a small breakfast (since lots of folks have no appetite when they wake up). So, you would then have a big lunch — much more so if you missed breakfast entirely or exercised in the morning. You will choose any meal as your largest meal of the day. It is all about finding out what works best for your body and lifestyle."

Myth: Fasting would make you incredibly stable and fit.

Fasting can do little in the short term.

Although intermittent fasting — when paired with adequate exercise — can aid in weight loss, those attempting the diet must keep in mind that following it alone is not a guaranteed path to fitness. I.F. is not a magical solution.

Maintaining good health and fitness is something you must strive at throughout your life — do not take it for granted. Fasting cannot provide you with your perfect body immediately. Even though you lose weight, you must sustain that by healthier activities such as a balanced diet and daily exercise.

Chapter 12.

INTERMITTENT FASTING FAQS

1. What Are the Consequences of Intermittent Fasting?

Transitioning to this way of eating is not pleasant for many people. According to a 2019 Nutrients study published in April, IF can cause migraines, dizziness, nausea, and insomnia. Additionally, it can make people feel hungry and weak in general, restricting their daily activity.

2. How Do I Manage Hunger When Fasting?

When your body transitions to IF, you are likely to feel hunger; experts say it will adapt. Through my personal observations and reviews from my patients, I have seen that it becomes easier. Thus, according to Harvard, IF does not enhance overall hunger. The 16:8 diet (or a combination thereof) appears to be the simplest for many people to incorporate into their daily lives without feeling deprived.

3. How Is Intermittent Fasting Different from Starvation?

However, according to Johns Hopkins hospital, IF is a form of feeding that involves switching between fasting (or a substantial decrease of calorie consumption) and eating at hours. It is unique from other diets in that it does not require the consumption of ingredients. IF is therefore not about deprivation. Other than that, it is about feeding within a set time period and fasting the remainder of the day and night.

4. Should Children Be Fasting?

Allowing your child to fast is almost certainly a bad idea.

5. Can Fasting Cause My Metabolism to Deteriorate?

Not at all. Short-term fasts have been shown to increase metabolism. However, prolonged fasts of three or more days have been shown to inhibit metabolism.

6. Is Fasting Associated with Muscle Loss?

All methods of weight reduction can result in muscle loss, which is why it is vital to lift weights and maintain a high protein intake. Intermittent fasting, according to one report, results in less muscle weakness than normal calories.

7. Can I Exercise When I am fasting?

Yes, exercises on an empty stomach are permissible. Certain individuals advocate for the use of branched-chain amino acids (BCAAs) prior to a fasted exercise.

8. Am I Allowed to Take Supplements During a Fast?

Yes. Bear in mind, however, that such supplements, such as fat-soluble vitamins, can function best when taken with meals.

9. Is not Skipping Breakfast Unhealthy?

Not at all. The issue is that many stereotypical breakfast-skippers lead unhealthy lives. If you make a point of eating nutritious food the rest of the day, the habit is completely safe.

10. Am I Allowed to Consume Liquids During Fast?

Of course. Tea, water and coffee, as well as other non-caloric drinks, are appropriate. Leave out the sugar in your coffee. Adding a small amount of cream or milk might be reasonable. Coffee is especially helpful during a fast, as it can help alleviate hunger.

11. Is Fasting Intermittently Expensive?

Intermittent fasting can cost no more than daily grocery shopping.

You are not required to be registered with any group. There are many 16:8 plans available online. The expense of the diet is entirely up to you, just as shopping is entirely up to you. Per week, you can spend less time eating over fewer time periods."

12. Is Interval Fasting Similar to Carb Cycling?

Carb spinning, when combined with extended fasting, can also help in weight loss.

Carb cycling is a metabolic method in which regular carbohydrate consumption is alternated. This is a popular technique used by bodybuilders and athletes and is the basis for the 5:2 diet. The reasoning is that when carbohydrate intake is limited, the body switches to fat as its main fuel supply, releasing ketone bodies. Generally, on low-carb days, fat consumption rises. And it is useful for more than just weight loss.

There is a substantial body of literature demonstrating that intermittent fasting increases cancer biomarkers, decreases oxidative stress, and improves cognitive function, with individuals losing up to 8% of their body weight in eight hours "weeks."

In the context of carb cycling, several trials have shown that a general decrease in calorie consumption improves well-being and increases longevity. However, carb cycling forces the body to use its fat reserves in order to burn stored fat.

13. Is Intermittent Fasting Worth Trying for Anyone Above the Age Of 50?

Yes. Intermittent fasting is certainly worth a try if you are in good health.

When combined with a nutritious diet and steps taken, intermittent fasting becomes a safe and simple way to boost one's health. While intermittent fasting is commonly considered effective for many healthy people, it is wise to communicate with your physician before attempting it. This is especially critical if you've any ongoing health problems, such as hypotension, diabetes, a history of disordered eating, or taking any medicine.

Even so, certain individuals should avoid intermittent fasting entirely. Intermittent fasting is often not advised for women who are breastfeeding, pregnant, or planning to conceive.

14. How Much Weight Can You Lose by Fasting Intermittently?

This is dependent on how much you limit the average calorie consumption. According to a 2014 analysis report, this eating pattern will result in a 4–9% weight loss over 4–26 weeks or 2-5kg for an individual weighing 70kg. The same study found that participants lost 5–7% of their waist circumference, showing a substantial reduction in unhealthy abdominal fat that accumulates across the organs and induces disease. Notably, clinical trial technology is also in its infancy.

15. If I Am Used to Snacking or Eating Every Few Hours, Would It Be Difficult for Me to Start an Intermittent Fasting Practice?

The first ten days of alternating day fasting or time-restricted eating routine are often the most difficult for first-time intermittent fasters. It usually takes people five fast days to become physically and mentally accustomed to experiencing regular energy levels on fast days. For the first ten days, however, many people can stick to their fast days or fasting times and work out as quickly when fasting as they can when feeding.

16. While Fasting, Would I Be Hungry?

Intermittent fasting has usually been found to have no discernible effect on ghrelin, the gut hunger hormone. It is natural to experience hunger while fasting, even after many

months of intermittent fasting. You can discover, though, that with experience, you become more adept at coping with hunger and distinguishing between genuine hunger and socially induced food cravings, for example. Consuming lots of calorie-free drinks or consuming up to 500 calories on a fast day will assist in managing hunger symptoms when fasting. IF has been shown in clinical studies to reduce leptin, a hormone that aids in energy expenditure control and increases post-meal satiety.

17. Are There Any Supplements That I Can Add to My Fasts to Increase Their Efficacy?

Today ketone ester supplements will help increase the blood ketone and achieve ketosis for mass consumption. These supplements can assist athletes in producing ketones, which can be beneficial as a source of energy during intense exercise. However, because you are still on a ketogenic diet, these supplements send conflicting messages to your body about whether it should be consuming fat or sugar for food. These supplements may not be beneficial or necessarily safe for long-term metabolic health.

18. How Long Would It Take to Arrive at Ketosis?

A condition of partial ketosis can take anywhere from 12 to 24 hours. When your serum glucose level decreases by 20% during a fast, your liver begins developing ketones to replace the energy your brain requires.

On a ketogenic diet, reaching complete ketosis will take up to ten days. Some people detect a fruity scent on their breath, a reduction in appetite, or lethargy as they undergo ketosis, although others feel none of these symptoms. To maintain a state of ketosis for an extended period, you must consume less than 30 grams of carbohydrates per day.

However, the metabolic effects of intermittent fasting do not include reaching a state of complete ketosis when fasting; insulin tolerance levels decline by up to 40% in stable obese people as they adhere to an IF protocol for only a few weeks.

19. Am I Permitted to Have Cheat Days?

It is vital to be adaptable. Intermittent fasting is best viewed as a way of life, not a trendy diet. IF expert advises people not to panic if they skip 2 or 3 fast days every month in their alternate day fasting tests. Occasionally, your fast days will fall on a holiday or another family occasion, and it might be more challenging to adhere to your fast rigidly than it is to eat a piece of cake.

Nevertheless, several people discover that "cheating" throws their whole fasting routine off track. If you become the kind of person who requires a great deal of structure to maintain a balanced lifestyle, experts advise against missing fast days for family activities or other special occasions. However, for many individuals, an odd cheat day would have no impact on their weight loss gains or metabolic fitness.

20. Is There an Optimal Manner to Break A Fast?

The effectiveness of various forms of meals before fast on metabolic well-being in humans has not been entirely tested in research studies.

A small number of current findings indicate that certain individuals may undergo an abrupt blood glucose spike correlated with insulin resistance, particularly in the high post-fast meal. However, severe postprandial insulin sensitivity can be more prevalent in unfamiliar persons with extended fasting cycles (16- to 24 hours). If you are fresh to fasting, you may need to end your overnight or extended fasts with meals that are low on the glycemic index and rich in fiber and plant fats (nuts, olives, seeds, coconut, avocado, etc.) For several months of prolonged fasting, the body's physiological response to a post-fast infusion of nutrients is likely to be altered. Over time, IF usually results in increased insulin sensitivity and decreased blood sugar levels.

21. IS ONE Form OF Intermittent FASTING MORE Efficient THAN ANOTHER?

Certain individuals will limit their feeding to an eight-hour duration, while others will rotate between a complete day of fasting and a day of regular eating. There is no form of intermittent fasting that is more reliable than another.

As with regular eating patterns, fasting should be individualized for each person and their habits. Certain individuals can handle true fasting through waking hours, while others function best with more regular meals.

22. How About the Notion That "Breakfast Is the Prime Meal"?

It is normal for participants to forego what we consider "breakfast" in order to adhere to the fast's time constraints. After all, the word "breakfast" applies to the meal that breaks our nighttime fast and supplies our bodies with sugar and other foods to power our metabolism. Breakfast has become synonymous with a meal that must be had first thing in the morning, though this is not always the case. When we feed, the consistency of the food we intake is far too important to our good health to ignore.

23. Is It Safe for Anyone to Try Intermittent Fasting?

Intermittent fasting is not advised for nursing mothers or pregnant women, adolescents/children, underweight people, the sick, or others with a history of disordered eating. Certain individuals on medication can benefit from the regular three meals a day after fast.

Additionally, it has been shown that intermittent fasting causes overall tiredness and hunger pains in its members. Certain individuals will find this so destructive that they may begin to

impact their way of life or feel alone as a result of being unable to participate in social activities that include food during fasts.

24. Will You Lose Weight by Eating the Same Amount of Food While Changing Your Eating Times?

Additional studies should be done to measure differences in fat mass between individuals that consume the same number of calories once during intermittent fasting and once while eating regularly. We must bear in mind that there are currently only a few human trials demonstrating intermittent fasting is mainly accountable for any of these related benefits and results. The experiments conducted so far have been short-term in nature, and the long-term results remain unknown.

We wish you luck if you decide to give it a shot and hope it works for you.

RECIPES

BREAKFAST

TURKISH FRIED EGGS, STRAINED YOGURT

Prep Time 15 Minutes | Cooking Time 10 Minutes | Servings 04

INGREDIENTS

- 2 ½ cups of Greek yogurt
- ½ teaspoon of coriander
- 1 tablespoon of parsley
- 1 pinch of tarragon
- 1 tablespoon of vegetable butter
- 4 Slices of bread
- 4 Large organic eggs
- ½ tablespoons of sundried tomato sauce
- 1 cup of goat cheese
- 1 tablespoon of sesame seed
- ½ teaspoon of sumac
- 1 pinch of salt and 1 pinch of pepper

DIRECTIONS

1. Rinse a paper towel thoroughly and wring it out well.
2. Open it over a bowl. Pour in the yogurt and let it drain, 1 hour, to obtain firm mixture
3. When the yogurt is completely drained, finely chop the cilantro, parsley and tarragon.
4. Add the salt and the pepper.
5. Mix your ingredients very well
6. Heat the butter in a non-stick pan.
7. Brown the slices of bread in it. Crack the eggs in a frying pan and cook them in the dish.
8. Spread each toast liberally with the yogurt mixture
9. Add the tomato sauce and a fried egg.
10. Crumble the goat cheese and sprinkle with sesame seeds and sumak.
11. Top with fresh herbs.
12. Serve and enjoy your breakfast!

NUTRITION

KCAL 112 PRO 9.1 CARB 12 FAT 8

BREAKFAST GRANOLA

Prep Time 10 Minutes | Cooking Time: 25 Minutes | Servings 3-4

INGREDIENTS:

- 3 ½ cups of oatmeal or buckwheat
- 2 cups of walnuts
- 2 ripe bananas
- 3 tablespoons of light cane sugar
- 1 cup of coconut oil
- 125 ml of agave syrup
- ½ tablespoons of cinnamon
- 1 rounded tablespoon of vanilla powder
- 1 tablespoon of cocoa powder

DIRECTIONS

1. Start by preheating the oven to 340 ° F.
2. Mix the dry ingredients (flakes, sugar, and cinnamon, vanilla, cocoa and nuts) in a bowl.
3. Then, in a saucepan, melt the coconut oil.
4. Having crushed the bananas beforehand, mix them with the coconut oil.
5. Then add the mixture in, along with the agave syrup (and dates and dark chocolate if you choose to add) and stir vigorously.
6. Spread the contents on a baking sheet and put in the oven
7. Bake for about 25 minutes.
8. Let cool, then break the granola and pour it into a jar.

NUTRITION

KCAL 140 PRO 3 CARB 14 FAT 9

SPINACH BREAKFAST WAFFLES

Prep Time 10 Minutes | Cooking Time   22 Minutes | Servings 4-6

INGREDIENTS

- 1 medium onion
- 1 tablespoon of olive oil
- 1 ½ cups of baby spinach
- 2 ¼ cups of all-purpose flour
- 1 tablespoon of baking powder
- 2 tablespoons of cornstarch
- 37 cl of buttermilk
- 1 tablespoon of vegetable oil
- 2 eggs; whites and yolks separated

- 1 cup of grated cottage cheese

For the topping:

- 2 cups of cherry tomatoes
- 2 eggs
- 1 handful of spinach
- 2 medium sliced into rings onions
- A few sprigs of parsley
- salt and pepper

DIRECTIONS

1. Peel and chop the onion; sauté in olive oil until translucent. Add the spinach and let reduce. Add the salt and the pepper.
2. In a bowl, combine the flour, baking powder, cornstarch and a pinch of salt.
3. In another bowl, combine the buttermilk, oil and egg yolks.
4. Gradually add the dry ingredients and mix until a smooth paste is obtained.
5. Mix the spinach with the grated cheese and pour everything into the dough.
6. Whip the egg whites; then gently fold them into the dough.
7. Oil a waffle iron and cook the waffles.
8. Preheat the oven to 360 ° F. Arrange the cherry tomatoes in a baking dish, sprinkle them with olive oil, salt and pepper. Bake for 15 minutes in a hot oven. Meanwhile, cook the eggs for 6 minutes in boiling water.
9. Place two waffles on each plate; divide the cherry tomatoes and spinach around them.
10. Add half an egg. Decorate with the young onions and a sprig of parsley.
11. Serve and enjoy your delicious waffles!

NUTRITION

KCAL 217 PRO 18 CARB 22 FAT 7

MIAMI FRUIT BOWL BREAKFAST

Prep Time 6 Minutes | Cooking Time: 0Minutes | Servings 2

INGREDIENTS:

- 1 half of a medium banana
- 2 tablespoons of rapeseed oil
- 2 tablespoons of crushed flax seeds and sesame seeds
- Half a lemon
- At least 3 different fruits: apple, peach, pear, kiwi, mango, papaya, strawberry, cherries, apricot, pineapple, grape, blueberry, persimmon, etc., but no citrus or dried fruits.
- 1 tbsp of 3 different oil seeds: squash seeds, walnuts, hazelnuts, macadamia nuts, almonds, etc.

DIRECTIONS

1. Mash the half a banana on a plate; then pour in two tablespoons of oil, mixing very well.
2. Squeeze the half lemon and add it to the preparation and incorporate your two tablespoons of your mixture of crushed seeds.
3. Then cut your fruit into small pieces and add them to the mixture, along with other oil seeds.
4. Your Yum is ready.
5. Serve and enjoy!

NUTRITION

KCAL 430 PRO 27 CARB 19 FAT 23

PRTOEIN BOWL BREAKFAST WITH GOJI BERRIES

Prep Time 10 Minutes | Cooking Time: 0 Minutes | Servings 3

INGREDIENTS:

- 1 kiwi
- 1 orange
- 1 handful of goji berries
- 1 handful of almonds
- 1 dash of raw cocoa nibs (crushed beans)
- 1 cup of plain soy yogurt
- 1 tablespoon of ground carob
- 1 banana
- 1 drizzle of maple syrup

DIRECTIONS

1. Start by crushing the banana, crushing the almonds coarsely and mixing the yogurt with the carob. Carob is a type of bean native to South America with a delicious taste reminiscent of caramel, cinnamon or hazelnut.
2. Pour the carob and banana yogurt on a plate; add the peeled and chopped kiwi, oranges, almonds and raw cocoa nibs then the goji berries
3. Arrange in a way you like
4. Serve and enjoy your protein breakfast

NUTRITION
KCAL 117 PRO 3 CARB 15 FAT 5.6

CHOCOLATE YOGURT BREAKFAST BOWL

Prep Time 10 Minutes | Cooking Time: 0 Minutes | Servings 2-4

INGREDIENTS:

- 1/2 very ripe persimmon
- A few raspberries
- 1 Clementine
- 1 handful of cashews which are an excellent source of protein
- 1 teaspoon of turmeric
- 2 pieces of dark chocolate, finely chopped
- Buckwheat petals
- 1 dash of maple syrup
- 1 pinch of raw cocoa
- 1 pinch of cinnamon
- 1 vegetable yogurt

DIRECTIONS

1. First mix the yogurt with the turmeric and then pour it into a small plate.
2. Roughly mix the persimmon with a pinch of cinnamon and pour it onto the plate with the yogurt.
3. Arrange the buckwheat, dark chocolate chips and fruit.
4. Sprinkle with raw cocoa powder, add maple syrup.
5. Serve and enjoy your Breakfast!

NUTRITION
KCAL 196.5 PRO 3 CARB 18.7 FAT 4

BREAKFAST MUESLI

Prep Time 10 Minutes | Cooking Time: 5 Minutes | Servings 2

INGREDIENTS:

- 2 Cups of whole almonds
- 1 tablespoon of pumpkin seeds
- 1 cup of whole wheat flour
- 2 tablespoons of maple syrup or honey
- ½ cup of nuts
- 1 Tablespoon of dark chocolate chips
- 1 cup of goji berries and or blackberries for vitamin C
- some raw cocoa beans

DIRECTIONS:

1. To make the base of this muesli, you need cereal flakes according to your tastes and flour (wheat, corn, etc.).
2. Mix the flakes in a bowl or container and lightly add the flour, maple syrup and oil, mix and bake for 5 minutes at 390 ° F.
3. Set aside; then add the dried fruits and oilseeds.
4. Add in the chocolate chips.
5. Mix everything.
6. Serve and enjoy your muesli

NUTRITION

KCAL 93 PRO 4 CARB 1.6 FAT 4

CHAKCHOUKA WITH KALE

Prep Time 10 Minutes | Cooking Time: 15 Minutes | Servings 4

INGREDIENTS:

- 4 organic eggs
- ½ pound of mushrooms
- 1 handful of kale
- 1 onion
- 1 garlic clove
- 1 cup of tomato sauce
- 1 cup of feta (crumbled)
- 1 tablespoon of olive oil
- 1 pinch of powdered cardamom
- 1 pinch of salt
- 1 pinch of pepper

DIRECTIONS:

1. Peel the onion and cut it into rings.
2. Peel and chop the garlic; then clean the mushrooms and cut them into slices.
3. Brown the onion and garlic in a saucepan with a little olive oil. Add the mushrooms and cook them briefly.
4. Add the tomato sauce; then season with cardamom powder, salt and pepper.
5. Let simmer for about 7 to 10 minutes
6. Crack the eggs in the pan and let them solidify at low temperature.
7. Meanwhile, blanch the cabbage in hot water before adding the rest of the preparation.
8. Crumble the feta on top.
9. Serve and enjoy your breakfast!

NUTRITION

KCAL304 PRO 14.2 CARB 23.1 FAT 18.1

MINI SPINACH PANCAKES

Prep Time 10 Minutes | Cooking Time: 10 Minutes | Servings 6

INGREDIENTS:

- ¼ Pound of baby spinach
- ½ pound of chickpeas (canned)
- 1 medium onion
- 2 large organic eggs
- ½ cup of milk
- 2 tablespoons of tahini
- 2 cups of flour
- 1 teaspoon of baking powder
- 1 tablespoon of olive oil
- 2 ½ cups of Greek yogurt
- 2 tablespoons of tahini
- 1 garlic clove
- ½ teaspoon of cayenne pepper
- sesame seeds (roasted)
- 1 pinch of salt and pepper
- Spinach chickpea

DIRECTIONS:

1. Finely chop the spinach in a blender, add the chickpeas and the young onion then mix to obtain a fluid texture.
2. Lightly beat the eggs and add the milk, tahini, flour and baking powder. Add the spinach and chickpeas. Add salt and pepper.
3. 3 Heat a pan with olive oil. Using a ladle, pour the dough in forming blinis and cook on both sides. Keep warm.
4. For the dip, mix the Greek yogurt with the tahini paste, the pressed garlic clove, cayenne pepper and salt.
5. Sprinkle with toasted sesame seeds, then serve and enjoy your breakfast!

NUTRITION

KCAL70 PRO 2 CARB 9 FAT 3

PASSION FRUIT GRANOLA BREAKFAST

Prep Time 10 Minutes | Cooking Time 30 Minutes | Servings 03

INGREDIENTS

- 1 mango
- 1 passion fruit
- ½ Pomegranates
- 50 peeled almonds
- 4 soy yogurts
- 1 Cup of sunflower seeds
- 1 Cup of walnut kernels
- 4 dates
- 1 teaspoon ground cinnamon

DIRECTIONS:

1. Chop the pitted dates with the almonds, sunflower seeds, walnuts and cinnamon until you have a very well combined mixture
2. Spread the mixture on baking paper, put in the oven at 110 ° F (th.2) and cook for 30 minutes.
3. Mix the mango into a fine purée, add the passion fruit.
4. Fluff the pomegranate. Divide the yogurt into 4 cups; place the mango compote on top, sprinkle with the crunchy mixture and pomegranate seeds.

NUTRITION

KCAL 345 PRO 10.1g CARB 45.3g FAT 13.9g

CINNAMON ROLLS BAKE

Prep Time 15 Minutes | Cooking Time: 20 Minutes | Servings 5-6

INGREDIENTS:

- 1 tablespoon of dry yeast
- 1 cup of milk (lukewarm)
- ½ teaspoon of salt
- 1 large egg
- 1 ½ pounds of flour
- 1 ¼ cups of butter
- 1 cup of brown sugar
- 1 cup of raisins
- ½ teaspoon of cinnamon powder
- 1 tablespoon of water
- 3 tablespoons of sugar
- 3 tablespoons of mascarpone

DIRECTIONS:

1. Dissolve the yeast in the milk and set it aside for 15 minutes.
2. Combine the salt, egg and flour. Gradually add the milk and knead to obtain smooth dough.
3. Form a ball, place it in a bowl and cover with a clean towel.
4. Let rest for 40 minutes; then on a floured surface, roll out the dough into a 50 x 60 cm rectangle
5. Melt the butter and add the brown sugar, raisins and cinnamon. Spread the mixture generously over the dough.
6. Roll the dough lengthwise to form a sausage. Press down on the last piece a little so that the roller does not open.
7. Cut the roll into 2.5 cm slices and place them on a baking sheet lined with baking paper. Cover with a towel and let stand for another 20 minutes.
8. Preheat your oven to a temperature of about 360 ° F.
9. Bake for 25 minutes in a hot oven or until the brioches are golden
10. Remove from the oven and let cool.
11. Mix the water and the icing sugar. Stir in the mascarpone. Brush the brioches with this mixture.
12. Serve immediately and enjoy your breakfast!

NUTRITION

KCAL309 PRO 11.6g CARB 44.5g FAT 3.8g

BREAKFAST CHIA PORRIDGE

Prep Time 10 Minutes | Cooking Time   10 Minutes | Servings 3

INGREDIENTS

- 1Cup of wheat semolina
- 2 Tablespoons of agave syrup
- 25 cl of semi-skimmed milk
- 1 juice of half a lemon
- 1 finely grated zest of a quarter of a lemon
- 1 vanilla pod
- 1 Cup of chia seeds
- 18 cl of almond milk
- 1 inch of finely chopped fresh ginger
- 2 Tablespoon of honey
- 2 Tablespoons of toasted flaked almonds
- 1 Orange, sliced

DIRECTIONS:

1. Combine all the ingredients in a saucepan (semolina, agave syrup, semi-skimmed milk, lemon juice, zest, seeds of a vanilla bean).
2. Bring the mixture to a boil, then lower the heat and cook for 3 or 4 minutes.
3. Let cool and chill in the refrigerator.
4. Then make the chia porridge. Mix all the ingredients in a bowl (chia seeds, almond milk, fresh ginger, honey), put in the refrigerator.
5. Leave to rest for at least an hour.
6. To serve, pour half the porridge into each bowl, then distribute the semolina
7. Sprinkle with almonds before placing the orange slices.

NUTRITION

KCAL 112 PRO 3.7g CARB 11.6g FAT 5.7g

BREAKFAST OATMEAL AND ZUCCHINI PANCAKES

Prep Time 10 Minutes | Cooking Time: 10 Minutes | Servings 2-4

INGREDIENTS:

- 4 thin slices of raw ham
- 1 Cup of oatmeal
- 100 ml of plain soy drink
- 2 eggs
- 1 zucchini
- 2 shallots
- 1 clove of garlic
- 10 basil leaves
- 2 tbsp of oil
- 1 Cup of olive
- 1 Pinch of herb salt
- 4 tbsp of squash seeds
- ½ melons

DIRECTIONS:

1. In a hollow container, place the oatmeal and pour in the plain soy drink. Mix and let the flakes rehydrate for 5 minutes then incorporate the 2 beaten eggs.
2. Meanwhile, finely slice the shallots in the direction of their fibers. Pour the olive oil in a non-stick pan, heat it gently and add the shallots with a few pinches of salt. Sauté them for 5 minutes, stirring often, until they are lightly colored and add them to the oatmeal.
3. Also add the grated zucchini without peeling it, the chopped garlic clove and the chopped basil.
4. Mix and adjust the salt; then roast the squash seeds in a dry pan for 10 minutes, stirring often; (they should not burn). Cut the melon into thin slices.
5. To cook the pancakes, pour a drizzle of olive oil in a non-stick pan and place 2 tablespoons of batter to form each pancake.
6. Cook them over low heat for about 5 minutes on each side and enjoy them with the melon slices, the cured ham and the pumpkin seeds.

NUTRITION
KCAL 84.5 PRO 4.3g CARB 16.6g FAT 1.2g

AVOCADO WAFFLES

Prep Time 15 Minutes | Cooking Time: 30 Minutes | Servings 4

INGREDIENTS:
For the waffles:

- 2 Cups of wheat flour
- 2 tablespoons of olive oil
- 1 Cup of brown rice flour
- 2 tablespoons of arrowroot
- 2 tsp of baking powder
- The Zest of a lemon
- 1 Cup of tahini

- 260 ml of soy milk

For the avocado whipped cream:

- 2 avocados
- 3 tsp lemon juice
- 1 tbsp of coriander
- 1 Cup of tofu
- 1 pinch of salt

INSTRUCTIONS:

1. Mix the flours with the cornstarch, baking powder, salt and lemon zest
2. Mix the tahini with the soy milk and pour over the flour and olive oil, while mixing vigorously to obtain a smooth and homogeneous mixture.
3. Set aside for about 30 minutes.
4. Bake in a waffle iron according to the manufacturer's instructions, greasing the waffle mold with a little olive oil.
5. Meanwhile, mix the avocado flesh for a long time with the silky tofu, salt and lemon juice, to obtain a smooth whipped cream texture.
6. Serve the waffles with the avocado whipped cream and sprinkle with fresh cilantro.
7. Serve and enjoy your waffles!

NUTRITION
KCAL 115 PRO 6 CARB 15 FAT 4.3

BREAKFAST PANCAKES

Prep Time 10 Minutes | Cooking Time: 10 Minutes | Servings 4

INGREDIENTS:

- 2 Cups of flour
- 2 Tablespoons of sugar
- 1 and ½ teaspoons of baking powder
- 1 Cup of melted margarine
- 325 ml of vegetable drink
- 1 pinch of salt
- 1 Cup of dark chocolate
- 1 orange (or any other seasonal fruit)
- 1 teaspoon of hazelnut paste (optional)

DIRECTIONS:

1. Combine all the dry ingredients in a bowl using a whisk.
2. Melt the margarine.
3. Add all the wet ingredients (margarine, vegetable drink) and mix again with a whisk until you get smooth, lump-free dough.
4. If the mixture seems too thick, add a little milk
5. Let the dough rest for ten minutes.
6. Meanwhile, zest with the orange then use 1/2 orange to make a juice
7. Cut the other half into slices.
8. Melt the chocolate in a saucepan with the orange juice. Once the chocolate is smooth, remove from the heat and add the hazelnut paste for a more delicious taste (option).
9. Heat a pancake pan and melt the margarine. Place a ladleful of batter in the hot pan, the pancake should be quite thin. Cook for about 1-2 minutes, then turn and cook for another 2 minutes.
10. Serve and place the chocolate inside, fold the pancakes into a triangle and add the orange zest and slices

NUTRITION

KCAL 183 PRO 9 CARB 12 FAT 8

BREAKFAST BANANA OATMEAL CRUSTED MUFFINS

Prep Time 10 Minutes | Cooking Time: 15 Minutes | Servings 6

INGREDIENTS:

- 1/4 cup mashed bananas
- 1/4 cup honey
- 1/2 tsp of almond extract
- 1 and 1/4 cups quick-cooking oatmeal
- 1/2 tsp of cinnamon
- 1/4 tsp of salt

DIRECTIONS:

1. Spray 6 cups or ramekins of a muffin pan with the vegetable oil.
2. In a bowl, combine the mashed bananas with the honey and the almond extract. In another bowl, combine the oatmeal with the cinnamon and salt; add to the previous mixture, stirring to moisten everything. Press this mixture at the bottom and on the edges of the muffin cups. Refrigerate for an hour or two.
3. Preheat the oven to 350 ° F (175 ° C).
4. Using your fingers, press the crusts to compact them well.
5. Bake for 10-12 minutes. Once out of the oven, press the crusts again with a spoon. Let cool.
6. Top with yogurt and berries

NUTRITION

KCAL 65.7 PRO 2.6g CARB 10.1g FAT 1.2g

BREAKFAST OATMEAL COOKIES

Prep Time 10 Minutes | Cooking Time: 10 Minutes | Servings 8

INGREDIENTS:

- 2 Tablespoons of vegetable oil
- 2 cups of oatmeal
- 1 cup whole wheat cake flour
- 1/4 cup ground flax seed
- 2 ½ tsp. 1/2 teaspoon ground Cinnamon
- 1/2 tsp of sea salt
- 1 teaspoon of baking soda
- 1 cup of honey
- 2 egg whites
- 4 tbsp of almond butter
- 1/2 tsp of vanilla extract
- ½ cup of semi-sweet (or dark) chocolate chips

DIRECTIONS:

1. Preheat the oven to 325 ° F (165 ° C). Lightly oil two cookie sheets.
2. In a large bowl, combine the oatmeal with the flour, ground flax seeds, cinnamon, salt and baking soda. Add honey, egg whites, almond butter and vanilla; mix until the dough is blended. Add the chocolate chips.
3. Shape the dough into 36 small balls and place them on the sheets.
4. Bake until cookies are golden, about 8-10 minutes. Let stand 10 minutes before transferring cookies to a wire rack.
5. Serve and enjoy your breakfast cookies

NUTRITION
KCAL 140 PRO 2 CARB 19 FAT 6

QUINOA BREAKFAST BOWL

Prep Time 10 Minutes | Cooking Time: 20 Minutes | Servings 3-4

INGREDIENTS:

- 1-1/2 cups of unsweetened pineapple juice
- 1 cup of coconut milk
- ½ teaspoon of ground cinnamon
- ¼ teaspoon of ground ginger
- 1 and ½ cups of rinsed quinoa
- 1 cup of drained crushed pineapple
- ¼ cup of packed brown sugar
- 1 cup of chopped peeled mango
- ½ cup of toasted chopped macadamia nuts
- ½ Cup of toasted sweetened shredded coconut

DIRECTIONS:

1. In a large saucepan, bring the pineapple juice, the coconut milk, the cinnamon and the ginger to a boil. Add the quinoa.
2. Reduce the heat; then let simmer, covered for about 15 to 20 minutes or until the liquid is completely absorbed.
3. Remove your mixture from the heat.
4. Stir in the pineapple; then add in the brown sugar.
5. Top with the mango and the macadamia nuts
6. Serve and enjoy with shredded coconut

NUTRITION
KCAL334.8 PRO 10.5g CARB 59.8 FAT 7.3g

BREAKFAST BANANA LOAF BREAD

Prep Time 15 Minutes | Cooking Time: 40 Minutes | Servings 5-6

INGREDIENTS:
- 1 ½ cups of wheat flour
- 100 ml of oat milk
- 100 ml of Vegetable oil
- 1 Cup of chocolate chips

DIRECTIONS:
1. Start by preheating your oven to 175 F°; then, mash the three bananas with a fork.
2. Add the agave syrup, vegetable oil and vegetable milk. Mix everything.
3. In a bowl, combine the flour, baking powder, ground almonds and cornstarch.
4. Pour in the banana mixture.
5. Add the chocolate chips and the crushed almonds.
6. Grease a loaf pan and pour the dough. Peel the last banana and cut it in half lengthwise. Place it on the cake as a topping
7. You can add a little quantity of almonds for topping
8. Finally, bake for about 35 to 40 minutes.
9. Serve and enjoy your bread!

NUTRITION
KCAL195.6 PRO 2.8g CARB 32g FAT 1.3g

OATMEAL BREAKFAST SQUARES

Prep Time 10 Minutes | Cooking Time: 25 Minutes | Servings 12

INGREDIENTS:
- 2 cups of old-fashioned oatmeal
- 1 cup of chopped walnuts
- 3/4 cup of brown sugar
- 3/4 cup of dried fruit
- ½ cup of all-purpose flour
- ½ cup whole wheat flour
- 1/2 cup toasted wheat germ (optional)
- 3/4 tsp. 1/2 teaspoon ground cinnamon
- 3/4 tsp. salt
- 1/2 cup vegetable oil
- 1/2 cup of honey
- 1 egg
- 2 tablespoons of teaspoon vanilla extract

DDIRECTIONS:
1. Preheat the oven to 350 ° F (175 ° C). Line a rectangle (13x9 inch) dish with parchment paper.
2. In a bowl, combine the oatmeal, walnuts, brown sugar, dried fruit, flour, wheat germ, cinnamon and salt.
3. Whisk oil with honey, egg and vanilla; add to bowl of dry ingredients and stir to moisten everything. Press everything into the baking dish.
4. Bake for 20-25 minutes. Let cool slightly before cutting into bars with a pizza wheel.
5. Serve and enjoy your breakfast !

NUTRITION
KCAL 153.2 PRO 3.6g CARB 26.3g FAT 4 g

CHOCOLATE WAFFLES

Prep Time 10 Minutes| Cooking Time: 10 Minutes| Servings: 3-4

INGREDIENTS:

- 2 Medium, separated eggs
- 1 and ½ Tablespoons of coconut flour
- 1 Tablespoon of cocoa, unsweetened
- 1 ½ Tablespoons of granulated Keto sweetener of choice or more, to your taste
- ½ Teaspoon of baking powder
- 1 Teaspoon of vanilla
- 1 and ½ Tablespoons of full fat milk or cream
- 1 Cup of melted butter

DIRECTIONS:

1. Start by whisking the egg whites until it becomes firm and until it forms a stiff peak
2. In a separate bowl, combine the egg yolk with the coconut flour, the sweetener and the baking powder
3. Add in the melted butter slowly and mix very well to ensure that you get a smooth consistency
4. Add in the vanilla and the milk and combine very well
5. Gently fold in spoons of the already whisked egg whites into the mixture of the yolk mixture.
6. Try to keep as much of the air as possible
7. Place enough of the mixture of the waffle into your already prepared warm waffle maker and cook until it becomes gold.
8. Serve and enjoy your delicious waffles!

NUTRITION
Kcal: 289 Fat: 26.6 Carbs: 7 Proteins: 7.2

OMELETTE

Prep Time 8 Minutes| Cooking Time: 8 Minutes| Servings: 3

INGREDIENTS

- 2 Tablespoons of butter
- 4 Medium eggs
- 4 Tablespoons of cream full fat
- Spices or herbs of your choice
- 1 Pinch of salt and pepper to taste

DIRECTIONS :

1. Whisk the eggs, the cream and the chosen herbs as well as the spices in a large bowl.
2. Melt the butter in the frying pan; then pour in the mixture of the burrito egg.
3. Swirl your frying pan until the mixture of the burrito mixture becomes evenly perfectly spread and thin
4. Cover the burrito with a lid and cook for about 2 minutes
5. Gently remove the burrito from your frying pan with a clean spatula to a clean plate.
6. Add your favorite toppings and fillings; then roll up the omelet
7. Serve and enjoy your breakfast!

NUTRITION
Kcal: 362 Fat: 31 Carbs: 1.5 Proteins: 21.5

SAUSAGE FRITTATA

Prep Time 10 Minutes| Cooking Time: 50 Minutes| Servings: 4-5

INGREDIENTS

- 12 Oz of raw breakfast sausage
- 1 Package of about 10 oz of thawed and drained frozen chopped spinach
- ½ Cup of crumbled feta cheese
- 12 Medium eggs
- ½ Cup of heavy cream
- ½ Cup of unsweetened milk
- ½ Teaspoon of salt
- ¼ Teaspoon of black pepper
- ¼ Teaspoon of ground nutmeg

DIRECTIONS :

1. Break the raw sausage up into pieces; then place raw sausage into small pieces and place it in a medium bowl.
2. Squeeze any remaining liquid out of the spinach; then break it up into the same bowl as the sausage.
3. Sprinkle the cheese on top of the mixture and toss very well until your mixtures is very well combined
4. Lightly spread the mixture into a greased casserole dish of about 13×9 casserole or into about 17 greased muffin cups
5. Meanwhile, in a large bowl; combine the eggs, the cream, the milk, the salt, the pepper, and the nutmeg all together until your mixture is fully combined.
6. Gently pour the mixture into the casserole or in the muffin cups about half ¾ way full.
7. Bake at about 375° F for about 50 minutes
8. Serve your breakfast warm or at room temperature.

NUTRITION

Kcal: 426 Fat: 36 Carbs: 21 Proteins: 21

DEVILED EGGS

Prep Time 10 Minutes| Cooking Time: 10 Minutes| Servings: 4

INGREDIENTS

- 2 Large hard boiled Eggs
- 1/8 Cup of Avocado Mayonnaise or of Mayonnaise
- ¼ Tablespoon of Dijon Mustard
- 1 Pinch of salt and 1 pinch of pepper to taste
- 1 Dash of Paprika for garnishing
- Chopped Green onion for garnishing

DIRECTIONS :

1. Peel the prepared eggs and slice it into halves.
2. Remove the egg yolks and place it into a bowl along with the avocado mayonnaise, the mustard, the salt, and the pepper.
3. Spoon the prepared filling into each of whites of the eggs and finish with the garnishes

NUTRITION

Kcal: 191 Fat: 18 Carbs: 7 Proteins: 5

FRENCH TOAST CASSEROLE

Prep Time 15 Minutes| Cooking Time: 45 Minutes| Servings: 4

INGREDIENTS

- ¼ bread loaf
- 1 ¼ Large Eggs
- ¼ Cup of heavy Cream
- 2 Tablespoons of Milk
- 1/8 Cup of Sukrin Gold
- ¼ Teaspoon of Vanilla Essence
- 1 Pinch of ground Cinnamon

Ingredients for the topping:

- ½ Tablespoons of Unsalted Butter
- ¼ Tablespoon of Sukrin Gold
- ¼ Teaspoon of Cinnamon ground

DIRECTIONS :

1. Preheat your oven to a temperature of about 390°F.
2. Cut the bread into large cubes; then add to a casserole dish of your choice.
3. In a bowl, add the cream; the eggs, the milk, the Sukrin gold, the vanilla, and the cinnamon; the whisk very well together.
4. Pour the prepared mixture over the already cubed bread and gently press down with a spoon and make sure that the bread soaks up the used liquid
5. In a separate bowl; add the ingredients of the toppings; then pour over the casserole dish and bake for about 30 to 45 minutes
6. Slice into about slices; then serve and enjoy your delicious French toast

NUTRITION

Kcal: 439 Fat: 42 Carbs: 7 Proteins: 10

CAULIFLOWER CORNED BEEF HASH

Prep Time 10 Minutes| Cooking Time: 8 Minutes| Servings: 3-4

INGREDIENTS :

- 1 Pound of Cauliflower; chopped into small florets
- 2 Tablespoons of Butter
- ½ Small of chopped onion
- 6 Ounces of roughly chopped corned Beef
- 1 Pinch of salt to taste
- 1 Pinch of pepper to taste

DIRECTIONS :

1. Start by the steam of the cauliflower until it becomes tender; then drain very well.
2. Place a large frying pan over a high heat; then add the onion and the butter and sauté until it becomes translucent.
3. Add in the cauliflower and sauté for about 4 to 5 minutes or until it starts to get brown
4. Continue cooking the cauliflower until it becomes brown
5. Season with 1 pinch of salt and 1 pinch of pepper
6. Serve and enjoy your breakfast!

NUTRITION

Kcal: 332 Fat: 25 Carbs: 12 Proteins: 17

BREAKFAST SAUSAGE PATTIES

Prep Time: 5 Minutes| Cooking Time: 10 Minutes| Servings: 3

INGREDIENTS :

- ½ Pound of ground pork, about 85% lean
- ½ Teaspoon of kosher salt
- ¼ Teaspoon of black pepper
- ¼ Teaspoon of dried thyme
- ½ Teaspoon of garlic powder
- ½ Teaspoon of smoked paprika
- ¼ Teaspoon of red pepper flakes
- 1 Pinch of cayenne pepper
- ½ Tablespoon of olive oil

DIRECTIONS :

1. In a bowl, use both your hands to mix the meat with the spices.
2. Form 2 patties of about ½ inch of thickness
3. Heat a large non-stick double-burner griddle and cook the patties for about 3 to 4 minutes and brush with the olive oil
4. Serve and enjoy your breakfast!

NUTRITION

Kcal: 200 Fat: 19 Carbs: 3 Proteins: 7

PANCAKES

Prep Time: 5 Minutes| Cooking Time: 10 Minutes| Servings: 3

INGREDIENTS:

- 1 Cup of flour
- 1 Tablespoon of Erythritol
- ¼ Teaspoon of baking powder
- 1 large egg
- 1/3 Cup of milk
- 2 Tablespoons of olive oil
- ½ Teaspoon of Vanilla extract
- 1 Pinch of sea salt

DIRECTIONS ;

1. Whisk all your ingredients all together in a large bowl until it becomes smooth.
2. Preheat a large oiled pan on the stove over a medium-low to a medium heat.
3. Drop the prepared batter into a prepared hot pan and form it into circles
4. Cover and cook for about 2 minutes; then flip and cook for about 1.5 minutes
5. Repeat the same process; then with the rest of the batter.

NUTRITION

Kcal: 268 Fat: 23 Carbs: 6 Proteins: 7

QUINOA BREAKFAST

Prep Time: 6 Minutes| Cooking Time: 15 Minutes| Servings: 3

INGREDIENTS:

- ½ Cup of rinsed and dry quinoa
- ¾ Cup of canned light coconut milk
- 2 Teaspoons of vanilla extract
- 1 and ½ teaspoon of cinnamon
- 1 Pinch of salt
- 1 Chopped banana
- 1/3 Cup of chopped and toasted pecans

DIRECTIONS:

1. Combine the quinoa, the coconut milk, the cinnamon and the vanilla in a medium saucepan and boil it.
2. Reduce the heat to a simmer and cover the saucepan for around 15 minutes
3. Divide the cooked quinoa in two bowls of your choice and cover it with pecans, bananas, and drops of coconut milk
4. Serve and enjoy your delicious and nutritious breakfast

NUTRITION

Kcal: 334 Fat: 7.3 Carbs: 54 Proteins: 10.5

SCRAMBLED EGGS WITH CHEESE

Prep Time: 6 Minutes| Cooking Time: 15 Minutes| Servings: 4

INGREDIENTS:

- 8 to 9 large eggs
- 1 tsp of Dijon mustard
- 1 pinch of kosher salt and 1 pinch of pepper
- 1 tbsp of olive oil or of unsalted butter
- 2 slices of thick-cut bacon, cooked and broken into small pieces
- 2 cups of spinach, torn
- 2 oz of shredded Gruyère cheese

DIRECTIONS:

1. In a large bowl, whisk all together the eggs with the Dijon mustard, about 1 tablespoon of water and about ½ teaspoon of salt and ½ teaspoon of pepper.
2. Heat the oil or the butter in about 10-inch non-stick skillet on a medium heat. Add in the eggs and cook while stirring with a rubber spatula every few seconds, to the desired doneness for about 2 to 3 minutes
3. Fold in the bacon, the spinach, and the Gruyère cheese.
4. Serve and enjoy your breakfast!

NUTRITION

Kcal: 133 Fat: 8 Carbs: 4 Proteins: 11

SOUP AND STEW RECIPES

LENTIL CREAM SOUP

Prep Time: 10 Minutes| Cooking Time: 10 minutes| Servings: 3-4

INGREDIENTS

- 6 cups of reduced-sodium chicken broth or of vegetable broth, divided
- 2 cups of rinsed dried lentils
- 1 to 2 bay leaves
- 1 clove, whole
- 1 medium chopped red onion
- 2 chopped celery ribs
- 2 tablespoons of butter
- 2 medium chopped carrots
- 1 teaspoon of salt
- 1 teaspoon of sugar
- ½ teaspoon of curry powder
- 1/8 teaspoon of pepper
- 2 Minced garlic cloves
- 3 cups of coarsely chopped fresh spinach
- 2 cups of heavy whipping cream
- 1 tablespoon of lemon juice
- 1/3 cup of minced fresh parsley

DIRECTIONS

1. In a large saucepan, combine about 4 cups of broth with the lentils, the bay leaf and the clove and bring to a boil.
2. Reduce the heat; then cover and let simmer until everything becomes tender for about 25 to 30 minutes
3. Meanwhile, in a Dutch oven, sauté the onion and the celery into the butter until it become crispy and tender at the same time
4. Add in the carrots, the salt; the sugar; the curry powder and the pepper; then sauté until the vegetables becomes tender for about 2 to 3 minutes
5. Add in the garlic; and cook for about 1 minute.
6. Drain the lentils; then discard the broth, the bay leaf and the clove. Add in the lentils to the vegetable mixture.
7. Add in the spinach, the remaining 2 cups of broth, the cream, the lemon juice and the parsley; then cook over a low heat for a few minutes
8. Serve and enjoy your soup!

NUTRITION

Kcal: 346 Fat: 20 Carbs: 29 Proteins: 13

BROCCOLI AND MUSHROOM SOUP

Prep Time: 10 Minutes| Cooking Time: 45 Minutes| Servings: 3-4

INGREDIENTS

- 1 bunch of broccoli of about 1 to ½ pounds
- 1 tablespoon canola oil
- ½ pound of sliced fresh mushrooms
- 1 tablespoon of reduced-sodium soy sauce
- 2 Finely chopped medium carrots
- 2 Finely chopped celery ribs
- ¼ cup of finely chopped onion
- 1 Finely minced garlic
- 1 carton of about 32 ounces of vegetable broth
- 2 Cups of water
- 2 tablespoons of lemon juice

DIRECTIONS:

1. Cut the broccoli florets into pieces of the bite-size peel and chop the stalks.
2. In a large saucepan, heat the oil over a medium-high heat; then sauté the mushrooms until they become tender for about 4 to 6 minutes.
3. Stir in the soy sauce; then remove from the pan; in the same pan, combine the broccoli stalks with the carrots
4. In the same pan, combine the broccoli stalks with the carrots, the celery, the onion, the garlic, the broth and the water; then bring to a boil and reduce the heat; then let simmer, uncovered for about 25 to 30 minutes
5. Puree the soup with an immersion blender; return to the pan; then stir in the florets and the mushrooms; and bring to a boil
6. Reduce the heat to a medium; then cook for about 8 to 10 minutes making sure to stir from time to time
7. Add in the lemon juice; then serve and enjoy!

NUTRITION

Kcal: 69 Fat: 3 Carbs: 35 Proteins: 4

SPLIT PEAS SOUP

Prep Time: 10 Minutes| Cooking Time: 8 Hours| Servings: 3-4

INGREDIENTS

- 1 package of about 16 ounces of rinsed dried green split peas
- 1 medium chopped leek (the white portion only)
- 3 chopped celery ribs
- 1 medium peeled and chopped potato
- 2 Chopped medium carrots
- 1 Minced garlic clove
- ¼ cup of minced fresh parsley
- 2 cartons of about 32 ounces each of reduced-sodium vegetable broth
- 1 and ½ teaspoons of ground mustard
- ½ teaspoon of pepper
- ½ teaspoon of dried oregano
- 1 to 2 bay leaves

DIRECTIONS

1. In a 5-qt. slow cooker; then combine all of your ingredients
2. Cover your slow cooker and cook on low for about 7 to 8 hours or until the peas become tender
3. Discard the bay leaf; and stir very well before serving it
4. Serve and enjoy your soup!

NUTRITION

Kcal: 248 Fat: 1 Carbs: 46 Proteins: 15

CELERY POTATO CHOWDER

Prep Time: 10 Minutes| Cooking Time: 15 Minutes| Servings: 4

INGREDIENTS

- 3 chopped celery ribs
- 2 finely chopped medium onions
- 3 chopped medium leeks (the white portion only)
- 1 medium chopped green pepper
- 6 Finely minced garlic cloves
- 2 tablespoons of olive oil
- 4 medium peeled and cubed potatoes
- 2 cans of about (14 and ½ ounces of each of vegetable broth
- ½ teaspoon of pepper
- ¼ teaspoon of salt
- ½ cup of coconut milk, optional
- 2 chopped green onions

DIRECTIONS

1. In a medium sized nonstick Dutch oven, sauté the celery with the onions, the leeks, the green pepper and the garlic into the oil until it becomes tender.
2. Add in the potatoes, the broth, the pepper and the salt and bring to a boil; then reduce the heat; cover and let simmer for about 10 to 15 minutes; stir from time to time
3. Puree the soup to the desired consistency with the help of a blender
4. Cool the soup; then puree in batches with the help of your blender; then sprinkle with the green onions
5. Serve and enjoy your soup!

NUTRITION

Kcal: 150 Fat: 4 Carbs: 27 Proteins: 3

BEAN AND FENNEL SOUP

Prep Time: 8 Minutes| Cooking Time: 25 Minutes| Servings: 3

INGREDIENTS

- 1 large; finely chopped onion,
- 1 small; thinly sliced fennel bulb
- 1 tablespoon of olive oil
- 5 Cups of reduced-sodium chicken broth or of vegetable broth
- 1 Can of 15 ounces of rinsed and drained cannellini beans
- 1 can of about 14 and ½ ounces of undrained diced tomatoes
- 1 teaspoon of dried thyme
- ¼ teaspoon of pepper
- 1 to 2 bay leaves
- 3 cups of shredded fresh spinach

DIRECTIONS

1. In a large saucepan, sauté the onion and the fennel into the oil until it becomes tender.
2. Add in the broth, the beans, the tomatoes, the thyme, the pepper and the bay leaf
3. Bring your ingredients to a boil; then reduce the heat; then cover and let simmer for about 30 minutes or until the fennel becomes tender.
4. Discard the bay leaf; then add in the spinach; then cook for about 3 to 4 additional minutes or until the spinach is wilted.

NUTRITION Kcal: 152 Fat: 3 Carbs: 23 Proteins: 8.1

CARROT SOUP

Prep Time: 10 Minutes| Cooking Time: 15 Minutes| Servings: 3

INGREDIENTS

- 1 medium, finely chopped onion
- 2 finely chopped celery ribs
- 1 tablespoon of canola oil
- 4 cups of vegetable broth
- 1 pound of sliced carrots
- 2 large peeled and cubed Yukon Gold potatoes
- 1 teaspoon of salt
- ¼ teaspoon of pepper
- Chopped fresh cilantro leaves

DIRECTIONS

1. In a large saucepan and over a medium high heat, sauté the onion and the celery into the oil until it becomes tender for about 2 minutes
2. Add in the broth, the carrots and the potatoes; then bring your soup to a boil
3. Reduce the heat; then cover and let simmer for about 15 to 20 minutes or until the vegetables become tender.
4. Remove the soup from the heat; then let cool slightly.
5. Transfer your soup to a blender; then cover and then process until it is very well blended and return to pan
6. Stir in the salt and the pepper; then heat through very well
7. Sprinkle with cilantro; then serve and enjoy your soup!

NUTRITION

Kcal: 176 Fat: 3 Carbs: 35 Proteins: 4

RICE SOUP

Prep Time: 6 Minutes| Cooking Time: 10 minutes| Servings: 3

INGREDIENTS

- 1 tablespoon of olive oil
- 3 Minced garlic cloves
- ¾ cup of uncooked arborio rice
- 1 carton of about 32 ounces of vegetable broth
- ¾ teaspoon of dried basil
- ½ teaspoon of dried thyme
- ¼ teaspoon of dried oregano
- 1 package of about 16 ounces of frozen broccoli-cauliflower blend
- 1 Can of about 15 ounces of rinsed and drained cannellini beans
- 2 Cups of fresh baby spinach
- Lemon wedges

DIRECTIONS

1. In a large saucepan, heat the oil over a medium heat; then sauté garlic for about 1 minute.
2. Add in the rice; then cook and stir for about 2 minutes.
3. Stir in the broth and the herbs; and bring to a boil; then reduce the heat; and let simmer, covered for about 10 minutes
4. Stir in the frozen vegetables and the beans; and cook while covered, over a medium heat for about 8 to 10 minutes
5. Stir in the spinach and serve with the lemon wedges
6. Enjoy your soup!

NUTRITION

Kcal: 303 Fat: 4 Carbs: 52 Proteins: 9

BROCCOLI SOUP

Prep Time: 5 Minutes| Cooking Time: 10 Minutes| Servings: 3

INGREDIENTS

- 1 tablespoon of canola oil
- 2 Finely minced garlic cloves
- 1 Package of 16 ounces of frozen broccoli florets
- 1 package of about 16 ounces of frozen cauliflower
- 5 cups of vegetable broth
- 2 teaspoons of curry powder
- ½ teaspoon of salt
- ½ teaspoon of pepper
- 1/8 teaspoon of ground nutmeg
- 1Cup of plain Greek yogurt, optional

DIRECTIONS

1. In a 6-qt. stockpot, heat the oil over a medium heat; then add in the garlic; cook and stir for about 1 minute
2. Add in the remaining ingredients except for the yogurt; then bring to a boil and reduce the heat; and let simmer, covered for about 8 to 10 minutes or until the vegetables become tender.
3. Remove the soup from the heat; then let cool slightly and process in a blender in batches
4. Return the pot to heat through
5. Top with the yogurt; then serve and enjoy your soup!

NUTRITION

Kcal: 84 Fat: 3 Carbs: 10 Proteins: 4

CARROT SOUP

Prep Time: 8 Minutes| Cooking Time: 25 Minutes| Servings: 3

INGREDIENTS:

- 2 medium, finely chopped carrots
- 1 small, finely chopped onion
- 2 tablespoons of olive oil
- 2 Minced garlic cloves
- 1 large peeled and cubed sweet potato
- ½ cup of chunky peanut butter
- 2 tablespoons of red curry paste
- 2 cans of about 14-1/2 ounces of vegetable broth
- 1 can of about 14-1/2 ounces of undrained fire-roasted diced tomatoes
- 1 to 2 bay leaves
- 1 to 2 fresh thyme sprigs
- ½ teaspoon of pepper
- ½ cup of unsalted peanuts

DIRECTIONS

1. In a large saucepan, cook the carrots and the onion into the oil over a medium heat for about 2 minutes. Add in the garlic; cook 1 minute longer.
2. Stir in the sweet potato; cook for about 2 minutes longer; then stir in the peanut butter and the curry paste
3. Add in the broth, the tomatoes; the bay leaf, the thyme and the pepper
4. Bring your mixture to a boil until everything is very well blended
5. Add in the broth, the tomatoes, the bay leaf, the thyme and the pepper.
6. Bring to a boil. Then reduce the heat; then cover and let simmer for about 15 to 20 minutes
7. Discard the bay leaf and the thyme sprig; then stir the soup until it is very well blended.
8. Sprinkle with the peanuts.

NUTRITION

Kcal: 276 Fat: 18 Carbs: 9 Proteins: 8

TORTILLA SOUP

Prep Time: 10 Minutes| Cooking Time: 15 Minutes| Servings: 3-4

INGREDIENTS

- 1 tablespoon of olive oil
- 1 medium, finely chopped onion
- 4 Finely minced garlic cloves
- 1 Seeded and chopped jalapeno pepper
- 8 cups of vegetable broth
- 1 cup of rinsed quinoa
- 2 teaspoons of chili powder
- ½ teaspoon of ground cumin
- ½ teaspoon of salt
- ¼teaspoon of pepper
- 1 can of about 15 ounces of rinsed and drained black beans
- 3 medium finely chopped tomatoes
- 1 cup of fresh or of frozen corn
- 1/3 cup of minced fresh cilantro
- Lime wedges
- Finely chopped cilantro

DIRECTIONS:

1. Heat the oil in your Dutch oven over a medium-high heat; then add in the onion, the garlic and the jalapeno pepper
2. Cook and stir for about 3 to 5 minutes; then add in the broth, the quinoa, and the seasonings. Bring your soup to a boil; then reduce the heat and let simmer, uncovered, until the quinoa is tender for about 10 minutes.
3. Add in the beans, the tomatoes, the corn and the cilantro; and let heat through
4. Serve with optional ingredients of your choice

NUTRITION

Kcal: 182 Fat: 4 Carbs: 31 Proteins: 7

POULTRY RECIPES

MAPLE CRANBERRY CHICKEN

Prep Time: 10 Minutes| Cooking Time: 20 Minutes| Servings: 4

INGREDIENTS

- 2 cups of fresh or frozen cranberries
- ¾ cup of water
- 1/3 cup of sugar
- 6 to 7 boneless skinless chicken breast halves of about 4 ounces each
- 1/2 teaspoon of salt
- ¼ teaspoon of pepper
- 1 tablespoon of canola oil
- ¼ cup of maple syrup

DIRECTIONS

1. In a small saucepan, combine all together the cranberriesb with the water and the sugar as wel
2. Cook over a medium heat until the berries pop, for about 15 minutes.
3. In the meantime; sprinkle the chicken with the salt and the pepper; then in a large nonstick skillet, cook the chicken into oil over a medium heat until the juices run clear for about 4 to 5 minutes per side.
4. Stir in the syrup into the cranberry mixture
5. Serve your chicken dish!

NURITION

Kcal: 236 Fat: 5 Carbs: 24 Proteins: 23

ROASTED CHICKEN LEGS

Prep Time: 15 Minutes| Cooking Time: 40 Minutes| Servings: 4-5

INGREDIENTS

- 4 to 5 pounds of chicken
- 2 teaspoons of kosher salt
- 1 teaspoon of coarsely ground pepper
- 2 teaspoons of olive oil
- 1 Dash of minced fresh thyme or rosemary

DIRECTIONS

1. Rub the outside of the chicken with the salt and the pepper; then transfer the chicken to a rack over a rimmed baking sheet.
2. Refrigerate while uncovered for an overnight.
3. Preheat your oven to a temperature of about 450°; then remove the chicken from the refrigerator while your oven heats up
4. Heat a cast iron of about 12-in or an ovenproof skillet into the oven for about 15 minutes.
5. Place the chicken on clear working surface, with the neck side down; then cut through with the skin where legs connect to the body
6. Press the thighs down so that the joints pop and the legs become flat.
7. Carefully place the chicken, with the breast side up, in a hot skillet; then press the legs down so that they lie flat onto the bottom of the pan.
8. Brush with the oil; then roast for about 35 to 40 minutes; then remove the chicken from the oven and set aside for about 10 minutes before serving
9. Top with the herbs before serving
10. Serve and enjoy!

NURITION

Kcal: 405 Fat: 24 Carbs: 6 Proteins: 44

PRESSURE COOKED CHICKEN WITH AVOCADO

Prep Time: 10 Minutes| Cooking Time: 35 Minutes| Servings: 4

INGREDIENTS

- 4lb of organic chicken
- 1 Tbsp of Coconut Oil
- 1 Teaspoon of paprika
- 1 and ½ cups of Pacific Chicken Bone Broth
- 1 Teaspoon of dried thyme
- ¼ teaspoon of freshly ground black pepper
- 1 teaspoon of ginger
- 2 Tbsp of lemon juice
- ½ Teaspoon of sea salt
- 6 cloves of peeled garlic
- 1 Avocado

DIRECTIONS:

1. In a medium bowl, combine the paprika, the thyme, the salt, the dried ginger and the pepper. Ten rub the seasoning over the outside of your chicken.
2. Heat the oil in your Instant Pot to simmering
3. Add the chicken breast with its side down and cook it for 6 minutes.
4. Now, flip your chicken and then add the broth, the lemon juice and the garlic cloves.
5. Lock the lid of your Instant pot and set the timer to 30 minutes at high pressure.
6. Meanwhile prepare the avocado cream by whisking the content of the avocado with 2 tbsp of coconut oil and ½ teaspoon of salt and salt.
7. Once the timer beeps, naturally release the pressure.
8. Remove your chicken from the Instant Pot and set it aside for around 5 minutes before serving it.
9. Serve and enjoy your Chicken dish!

NURITION

Kcal: 373.6 Fat: 19.8 Carbs: 8.8 Proteins: 40.8

PRESSURE-COOKED CHICKEN WITH ALMONDS

Prep Time: 10 Minutes| Cooking Time: 20 Minutes| Servings: 4

INGREDIENTS:

- 3 to 4 boneless and skinless chicken breasts
- 2 Tbsp of chicken seasoning
- 1tbsp of fresh ginger
- ¼ Cup of coconut oil
- 3 Tbsp of lime juice
- For the Salsa of the Mango Pepper: 2 cups of diced fresh mangos + 1 cup of diced red bell pepper + 3 tbsp of minced red onion + 1 tbsp of lime juice + 2 Tbsp of minced fresh cilantro +1 pinch of salt + 1 pinch of pepper to taste

DIRECTIONS:

1. Place your Instant Pot on a medium high heat and pour 2 cups of water into it
2. Place the trivet or the steaming basket in the Instant Pot
3. Trim the excess quantity of fat from your chicken, rinse it and pat dry it; if you need to. Cut the chicken into cubes
4. Place your chicken into a plastic bag and add the seasoning to it; the oil and the lemon juice. Then seal the bag.
5. Once you placed the chicken in the steaming basket, close the lid and press the steam feature on a high pressure for 10 minutes.
6. Meanwhile, combine the ingredients of the mango salsa and season it with oil, salt and pepper.
7. Once the timer beeps, make a quick release of pressure and serve your chicken with mango salsa, sprinkle almond halves; enjoy!

NURITION

Kcal: 431 Fat: 13 Carbs: 49 Proteins: 32

CHICKEN CORDON BLEU

Prep Time: 10 Minutes| Cooking Time: 27Minutes| Servings: 5

INGREDIENTS

- 1 tube of about 13.8 ounces of refrigerated pizza crust
- 4 thin slices of deli ham
- 1 and 1/2 cups shredded cooked chicken
- 6 slices of Swiss cheese
- 1 tablespoon of melted butter
- 1 Optional roasted garlic Alfredo sauce

DIRECTIONS

1. Preheat your oven to a temperature of about 400°F. Unroll the pizza dough onto a clean baking sheet; then layer with the ham, the chicken and the cheese to within about ½ inch of edges
2. Roll up the jelly-roll style, making sure to start with the long side; then pinch the seam to seal and tuck the ends under.
3. Brush with the melted butter; then bake until the crust becomes dark golden brown for about 18 to 22 minutes
4. Let stand for about 5 minutes before slicing your cordon bleu; then slice
5. Serve and enjoy with the Alfredo sauce!
6. If desired, serve with Alfredo sauce for dipping.

NURITION

Kcal: 298 Fat: 10 Carbs: 32 Proteins: 21

BUTTERED PRESSURE-COOKED CHICKEN

Prep Time: 15 Minutes| Cooking Time: 20 Minutes| Servings: 4

INGREDIENTS:

- 9 boneless and skinless chicken thighs
- 2 cups of diced tomatoes with its juice
- 3 Seeded and chopped jalapeno peppers
- 2 Tbsp of peeled and chopped fresh ginger root
- ½ Cup of unsalted butter
- 2 Teaspoons of ground cumin
- 1 Tbsp of paprika
- 2 Teaspoons of kosher salt
- ¾ Cup of heavy cream
- ¾ Cup of Greek yogurt
- 2 Teaspoons of Garam Masala
- 2 Teaspoons of ground roasted cumin seeds
- 2 Tbsp of cornstarch
- 2 Tbsp of water
- ¼ Cup of minced cilantro

DIRECTIONS:

1. Cut the chicken into cubes or quarters. Put the tomatoes, the jalapeno and the ginger into a food processor and blend all of the ingredients.
2. Add a little bit of butter to the Instant Pot, select the sauté function.
3. When the butter is completely melted, add the chicken and cook for 3 minutes.
4. Remove the chicken into a bow and set it aside.
5. Add the ground cumin and the paprika to the butter into your Instant Pot and cook all together for 1 minute.
6. Add the tomatoes, the salt, the cream, the yogurt and the chicken.
7. Stir and cover the lid of the Instant Pot; then set high pressure for around 5 minutes.
8. When the timer beeps, naturally release the pressure for around 10 minutes.
9. Add the Garam Masala and the roasted cumin and combine the ingredients together; then press sauté to boil for 3 minutes.
10. Serve and enjoy with rice and garnish with cilantro.

NURITION

Kcal: 355 Fat: 23 Carbs: 14 Proteins: 23

INSTANT POT CHICKEN BREAST

Prep Time: 15 Minutes| Cooking Time: 20 Minutes| Servings: 4

INGREDIENTS

- 1-2 pounds of chicken breasts or thighs
- 1 teaspoon sea salt
- 1 onion, diced
- 1 tablespoon avocado oil, lard, or ghee
- 5 garlic cloves, minced
- 1/2 cup organic chicken broth or homemade
- 1 teaspoon dried parsley
- 1/4 teaspoon paprika
- 1 large lemon juiced
- 3-4 teaspoons (or more) arrowroot flour

DIRECTIONS:

1. Turn your Instant Pot onto the sauté feature and place in the diced onion and cooking fat
2. Cook the onions for 5-10 minutes or until softened. You can also choose to cook until they start to brown
3. Add in the remaining ingredients except for the arrowroot flour and secure the lid on your Instant Pot
4. Select the "Poultry" setting and make sure your steam valve is closed
5. Allow the cooking time to complete, release steam valve to vent and then carefully remove lid
6. At this point you may thicken your sauce by making slurry
7. To do this remove about 1/4 cup sauce from the pot, add in the arrowroot flour, and then reintroduce the slurry into the remaining liquid
8. Stir and serve right away. This also reheats well as leftovers

NURITION
Kcal: 170 Fat: 6 Carbs: 1 Proteins: 25

PRESSURE-COOKED CHICKEN DRUMSTICKS

Prep Time: 10 Minutes| Cooking Time: 90 Minutes| Servings: 5

INGREDIENTS

- 2 bone-in Chicken Breasts
- 2 tablespoons Organic Grass-Fed Butter ghee or coconut oil
- 1 teaspoon chili powder
- 2 teaspoons cumin
- 1 pinch Crushed Red Pepper Flakes
- 1 1/2 teaspoons Sea Salt
- 1/2 teaspoon Organic White Pepper
- 1 teaspoon Organic Garlic Powder
- 1 teaspoon Organic Onion Powder
- 1/2 large Organic Yellow Onion chopped
- 2 ribs celery chopped
- 1/2 green pepper chopped
- 1/2 red pepper chopped
- 4 cups Water, filtered
- 2 tablespoon potato starch
- 1 cup organic coconut milk

DIRECTIONS:

1. Liberally season the chicken breasts with the seasoning.
2. In a large Dutch oven or heavy bottomed pot, heat butter over medium heat. Place chicken breasts, skin side down in pot and lightly brown (2-3 minutes)
3. Turn chicken breasts over (bone side down); add onions, celery and peppers.
4. Sauté until soft, 2-3 minutes.
5. Add water bring to a simmer. Cover and turn heat to low and cook for 1 hour.
6. Remove chicken breasts from liquid, allow to cool
7. Remove skin and bones (discard or freeze use in bone broth next time you make it) roughly chop or shred chicken meat and add back into soup.
8. In a small bowl or cup, whisk together potato starch and about 1/4 cup of the liquid from the soup until smooth. Add into the soup and stir well to combine.
9. Allow thickener to cook in for 2-3 minutes then turn off heat and stir in coconut milk.
10. Serve in bowls topped with chunks of avocado. It is also delicious served overtop of rice

NURITION
Kcal: 226 Fat: 8 Carbs: 19.6 Proteins: 19.72

CHINESE-STYLE CHICKEN

Prep Time: 10 Minutes| Cooking Time: 10 Minutes| Servings: 4

INGREDIENTS

- 1 pound boneless skinless chicken breasts, sliced into strips
- 1/2 cup chicken broth
- 1/4 cup coconut aminos
- 2 tablespoons sesame oil
- 1 teaspoon fish sauce
- 1 1-inch knob ginger, crushed
- 2 cloves garlic, minced
- 1/4 teaspoon fine sea salt
- 1/4 teaspoon black pepper
- Optional: red pepper flakes, as desired
- 1/4 teaspoon apple cider vinegar
- 10-12 ounces of broccoli florets, about 5-6 cups
- Sesame seeds, for garnish
- Slurry:
- 2 tablespoons arrowroot or tapioca flour
- 2 tablespoons water

DIRECTIONS:

1. Place chicken in the insert of your Pressure Cooker/Instant Pot.
2. Add in broth, coconut aminos, sesame oil, fish sauce, ginger, garlic, salt and pepper.
3. Cook on manual, high pressure for 8 minutes.
4. Turn the knob to quick release.
5. Add in the slurry and mix to combine.
6. Press off, and then turn on the sauté function. Add in the broccoli on sauté for about 5 minutes, stirring often, or until broccoli has softened and sauce has reduced slightly and thickened. Add apple cider vinegar and mix (this won't add any vinegar taste, just brings out the flavor in the sauce).
7. Garnish and enjoy.
8. Serve with cauliflower rice or white rice!

NURITION

Kcal: 190 Fat: 4 Carbs: 6 Proteins: 36

CHICKEN MASALA

Prep Time: 10 Minutes| Cooking Time: 20 Minutes| Servings: 4

INGREDIENTS

- 1 1/2 tablespoons olive oil
- 1 small onion, finely diced
- 3 cloves garlic, minced
- 1 (2-inch) piece fresh ginger, peeled and grated
- 1/2 cup chicken broth, divided
- 1 1/2 tablespoons Garam Masala
- 1 teaspoon smoked paprika
- 1/2 teaspoon ground turmeric
- 1/2 teaspoon kosher salt
- 1/4 teaspoon cayenne pepper (optional)
- 1 1/2 pounds boneless, skinless chicken thighs, cut into 1 1/2-inch pieces
- 1/2 cup coconut milk
- Fresh cilantro, chopped

DEIRECTIONS:

1. Sauté the aromatics; then set an electric pressure cooker to the sauté feature.
2. Add in the oil and heat until shimmering but not smoking.
3. Add the onion and sauté until softened, about 3 minutes. Add the garlic and ginger and cook until soft and fragrant. The mixture might stick a little to the bottom of the pot; this is normal.
4. Deglaze and add spices: Add 1/4 cup of the chicken broth. Cook, gently scraping the bottom of the pot with a wooden spoon to loosen any stuck-on bits, until the chicken broth reduces by half. Add the Garam Masala, paprika, turmeric, salt, and cayenne pepper, and stir to combine.
5. Add the chicken, broth
6. Add the chicken and stir to combine. Add the remaining 1/4 cup of chicken broth
7. Pressure-cook: Close and lock lid. Pressure-cook for 10 minutes at HIGH pressure. When cooking time is complete, do a quick release of the pressure.
8. Add the creamy element
9. Stir the coconut milk into the sauce.
10. Top with chopped cilantro.

NURITION

Kcal: 358 Fat: 14.8 Carbs: 32.5 Proteins: 18.8

BEEF

BEEF DISH WITH GARLIC AND PARSLEY

Prep Time: 10 Minutes| Cooking Time: 10 Minutes| Servings: 3

INGREDIENTS:

- ½ Pound of sirloin steak cut into small chunks
- ½ Tablespoon of olive oil
- 1 Tablespoons of almond butter or coconut oil
- 1 Teaspoons of minced garlic
- 1 Pinch of salt
- 1 pinch of pepper
- ½ Tablespoon of minced parsley

DIRECTIONS:

1. Start by heating the olive oil in a large pan over a medium high heat; then season with the salt and the pepper to taste
2. Put the steak in the pan in one single layer; then cook for about for about 3 to 4 minutes
3. Add the almond butter and the garlic to the pan and cook for about 1 to 2 minutes, and stir very well
4. Sprinkle with parsley; then serve
5. Enjoy your dish!

NURITION

Kcal: 272 Fat: 15 Carbs: 10 Proteins: 31

MONGOLIAN BEEF

Prep Time: 10 Minutes| Cooking Time: 9 Minutes| Servings: 4

INGREDIENTS:

- ½ Pound of sliced flank steak into stripes
- 1 Tablespoons of olive oil, divided
- ½ Tablespoon of peeled and grated fresh ginger
- 1 Minced garlic clove
- 1 Tablespoons of coconut aminos
- ¼ Cup of water
- 1/3 Cup of So Nourished Erythritol
- ½ Teaspoon of red pepper flakes
- 1 Teaspoon of xanthan gum
- 1 Pinch of salt
- 1 Pinch of pepper
- 1 Sliced scallion

DIRECTIONS:

1. In a large saucepan; heat half of the olive oil; then add the minced garlic and the grated ginger and fry for about 30 seconds.
2. Add the water, the coconut aminos, the erythritol, the red pepper flakes and let simmer on a high heat for about 3 to 4 minutes.
3. Turn off the heat and set aside.
4. Add the xanthan gum and the beef strips to a zip bag and toss very well.
5. In a large frying pan, heat the other half of the olive oil until it becomes hot.
6. Add in the beef strips and fry stir for several minutes
7. Heat a pan over a medium high heat; then add the sauce and the beef
8. Add 1 pinch of salt and 1 pinch of pepper; then cook for about 1 minute
9. Divide between two plates
10. Serve and enjoy your dish!

NURITION

Kcal: 233 Fat: 13 Carbs: 3 Proteins: 25

STUFFED FLANK STEAK

Prep Time: 10 Minutes| Cooking Time: 9 Minutes| Servings: 4

INGREDIENTS:

- ½ Pound of butterflied flank steak
- 1 Cup of fresh baby spinach
- 1/3 Cup of crumbled feta cheese
- 1/3 Cup of chopped sun and packed in olive oil, dried tomatoes packed in olive oil, drained very well
- 1 Minced garlic clove
- ¼ Teaspoon of dried basil
- 1 Pinch of fresh ground pepper
- 1 Tablespoon of pasta tomato, divided
- ½ Tablespoon of olive oil
- 1 Pinch of salt
- 1 Pinch of fresh ground pepper
- Chopped fresh parsley

DIRECTIONS :

1. Preheat your oven to a temperature of 400°F.
2. With a sharp knife, butterfly the beef steak by placing your hand right on top of the meat and then cutting in an horizontal way into the steak just about 1 inch before cutting the meat into 2 separate pieces
3. Open up the beef steak and set it aside.
4. In a large mixing bowl, combine the chopped spinach with the cheese, the sun dried tomatoes, the garlic, the basil and the fresh ground pepper and mix very well until your ingredients are very well incorporated.
5. Spread about 1/3 cup of tomato sauce on top of the steak and top with the already prepared mixture of the spinach
6. Roll up the steak and secure it with the Kitchen twine
7. Brush your stuffed flank steak with the olive oil and season it with the salt and the pepper.
8. Spread the rest of the sauce of tomato on top and around the edges
9. Transfer to a baking dish; then bake for about 35 to 40 minutes
10. Remove from the oven and transfer the steak to a cutting board.
11. Let your stuffed steak rest for about 10 minutes right before removing the kitchen twine
12. Remove the kitchen twine; then slice the stuffed steak into rounds of about ¼ inch each
13. Spoon the tomato sauce from the baking dish over the rounds, and top with the fresh parsley
14. Serve and enjoy your dish!

NURITION

Kcal: 349 Fat: 13 Carbs: 3 Proteins: 25

BEEF MEATLOAF

Prep Time: 10 Minutes| Cooking Time: 60 Minutes| Servings: 5

INGREDIENTS:

- ½ Pound of grass-fed ground beef
- ½ Diced onion
- 1 Cup of cooked sweet potato
- 2 Tablespoons of almond flour
- 1Tablespoon of coconut flour
- 1 Large egg
- 1 Tablespoon o gluten-free ketchup
- 1 Tablespoon of coconut aminos
- 1 Pinch of salt
- 1 Minced garlic clove Teaspoon

For the glaze

- ¼ Cup of gluten free ketchup
- 1 Tablespoons of coconut aminos
- 1 Tablespoon of erythritol

DIRECTIONS:

1. Preheat your oven to about 350°F and prepare a baking tray by lining it with a cookie sheet or a parchment paper
2. Put the diced onion with a little bit of coconut oil in a saucepan; then sauté it until it becomes soft for about 6 minutes
3. In a large and deep bowl; mix altogether the beef, the onion, the sweet potato, the almond flour, the coconut flour, the egg, the ketchup, the coconut aminos, the salt, and the garlic powder together.
4. Make the form of a loaf and put it into a pan; then mix all the ingredients of the glaze in a bowl and pour it over the meatloaf
5. Bake your meatloaf for about 60 minutes; then remove it from the oven.
6. Set the meatloaf aside to cool; then slice it, serve and enjoy it!

NURITION

Kcal: 471 Fat: 15.3 Carbs: 3.9 Proteins: 17.4

ITALIAN-STYLE BEEF STEAK

Prep Time: 15 Minutes| Cooking Time: 30 Minutes| Servings: 2-3

INGREDIENTS:

- ½ Pound of Flank Steak
- ¼ Pound of diced Bacon
- ½ Cup of chopped Mushrooms
- 2 Oz of Baby Spinach
- 1 Tablespoon of Parsley
- 1 Minced Garlic Clove
- 1 Pinch of salt
- 1 Pinch of fresh black pepper

DIRECTIONS :

1. Preheat your oven to a temperature for about 400° F
2. Arrange the bacon in an oven-proof tray
3. Drizzle the bacon with a little bit of coconut oil; then place the tray in the oven
4. Bake the bacon for about 8 to 10 minutes.
5. Remove the tray from the oven; then in another pan; sauté your mushrooms with the seasonings
6. Add the spinach into the pan and stir your ingredients
7. Lay the flank down; then spread the spinach mixture over the steak
8. Roll the flank steak and the spinach with a twine
9. Heat up a skillet over a medium high heat and pour 1 tablespoon of oil in it
10. Sear the steak into the skillet for about 25 minutes
11. Remove the meat from the skillet and set it aside to cool for about 5 minutes
12. Serve and enjoy your dish!

NURITION

Kcal: 386 Fat: 30 Carbs: 3 Proteins: 23

BEEF CURRY

Prep Time: 10 Minutes| Cooking Time: 15 Minutes| Servings: 4

INGREDIENTS:

- 1 Tablespoon of Oil
- ½ Pound of diced Beef
- 2 Tablespoons of yellow Curry Paste
- 2 Kaffir Lime Leaves
- 1 Pinch of salt
- 1 Tablespoon of Lime Juice
- 3.5 Oz of Coconut Cream
- 1 Teaspoon of Erythritol optional

DIRECTIONS :

1. Chop the beef if you have bought rump steak or gravy steak; then place it in a large frying pan over a medium high heat with about 1 tablespoon of oil
2. Sear the beef chunks for about 5 minutes; then add the yellow curry paste, the coconut cream, the kaffir lime leaves
3. Add in the coconut cream; the yellow curry paste, the Kaffir lime leaves and cook for about 10 minutes on a low heat
4. Add in the salt, the lime juice and the erythritol, and mix all together very well.
5. Serve with the Riced Cauliflower
6. Enjoy your dish!

NURITION
Kcal: 620 Fat: 48 Carbs: 14 Proteins: 40

BEEF STEAK WITH GREEN PEPPER

Prep Time: 8 Minutes| Cooking Time: 20 Minutes| Servings: 2-3

INGREDIENTS:

- ½ Pound of thinly stripped sirloin steak
- 1 Tablespoons of olive oil
- 3 Thinly sliced mini sweet peppers
- 1 Diagonally sliced scallions
- 1Tablespoon of minced fresh ginger
- 1Minced garlic clove

To make the marinade
- ¼ Cup of coconut aminos
- ⅓ Cup of water
- 2 Tablespoons of white wine vinegar
- ¼ Teaspoon of fresh coarse ground black pepper

DIRECTIONS:

1. Combine the ingredients of the marinade into a large bowl
2. Add the thinly sliced steak to your marinade; then toss your ingredients very well to coat it
3. Refrigerate your marinade for about 15 minutes
4. Add some coconut oil to a large skillet and place it over a medium heat
5. Add the white parts of the scallions, the bell peppers, the ginger, and the garlic for about 4 minutes
6. Transfer your ingredients to a plate
7. Take the steak out of the marinade; then add it to your skillet and sauté it for about 4 minutes

NURITION
Kcal: 337.3 Fat: 23.4 Carbs: 23.4 Proteins: 17.3

BEEF PIE

Prep Time: 15 Minutes| Cooking Time: 40 Minutes| Servings: 5

INGREDIENTS:

- ¼ Pound of finely grass-fed ground beef
- 1 Finely chopped garlic clove
- 1 Finely chopped small red onion
- 1 Teaspoon of dried oregano
- 1 Teaspoon of dried thyme
- ½ Teaspoon of dried tomato mix
- 1 Tablespoon of chopped fresh parsley
- ¼ Tablespoon of tomato puree
- ½ Tablespoon of extra virgin olive oil
- 1 Pinch of salt
- 1 Pinch of pepper
- 2 quality beef sausages
- 3 Cherry tomatoes
- 1 Tablespoon of dried oregano
- 1 Tablespoon of extra virgin olive oil
- 1 Handful of mushrooms (Shiitake mushrooms)
- 2 Large eggs
- 1 Pinch of salt
- 1 Pinch of pepper
- Some fresh basil leaves for garnishing

DIRECTIONS ;

1. Preheat your oven to a temperature of about 380° F
2. Roast your sausages into the oven for about 20 minutes
3. Combine all of your ingredients altogether; then transfer it into a lightly greased sandwich tin.
4. Spread the mixture of the meat into the base of the tin; then press it to the bottom and make the sides up to make the crust
5. Bake in the oven for about 20 minutes
6. In the meantime; slice the tomatoes into halves; then arrange it over a baking tray; then drizzle with a little bit of oil, 1 pinch of salt, 1 pinch of pepper and oregano
7. Roast the tomatoes in the oven for about 10 minutes
8. Once your base is perfectly cooked and the sausages are cooked too, slice into halves
9. Crack the eggs into a bowl; then whisk it and season it with 1 pinch of salt and 1 pinch of pepper
10. Pour the eggs right over the top of the base of the meat
11. Arrange the halves of the sausages, the tomatoes, the shiitake and the mushrooms over the top and bake it into the oven for about 20 minutes
12. Add 1 fried egg to your dish and garnish with fresh basil
13. Serve your pie and enjoy its delicious taste!

NURITION

Kcal: 570.7 Fat: 51 Carbs: 1.5 Proteins: 25.4

BEEF CHILI

Prep Time: 8 Minutes| Cooking Time: 35 Minutes| Servings: 3

INGREDIENTS:

- 1 Pound of beef meat
- ¼ Chopped red onion
- ¼ Teaspoon of minced garlic
- 2 Tablespoons of tomato sauce
- 1 Cup of roughly diced tomatoes with the juice
- 1 Cup of beef stock
- ½ Cup of sliced carrots
- 1 Cups of peeled and diced sweet potato
- 1 Bay leaf
- ½ Teaspoon of thyme
- 1 Pinch of salt
- 1 Pinch of black pepper
- ½ Cup of chili powder
- 1 Pinch of oregano
- 1 Pinch of red pepper flakes

DIRECTIONS :

1. In a large and deep saucepan, sauté the beef meat with the onions and the garlic into 1 tablespoon of coconut oil
2. Drain off any fat from the pan; then add the rest of your ingredients and mix very well
3. Let your ingredients boil for about 35 minutes over a low heat or until the vegetables become tender.
4. Remove; the bay leaves
5. Serve and enjoy your chili!

NURITION

Kcal: 367.8 Fat: 26.9 Carbs: 5.5 Proteins: 24.8

GROUND BEEF AND CAULIFLOWER TRAY

Prep Time: 15 Minutes| Cooking Time: 30 Minutes| Servings: 4

INGREDIENTS:

- ½ Pound of ground meat
- ½ Cup of chopped cauliflower
- 1 Teaspoon of steak seasoning
- ¼ Cup of shredded cheddar cheese
- ½ Tablespoon of extra virgin olive oil
- 2 Oz of cream cheese, chopped into cubes
- 1 Egg
- ¼ Cup of heavy cream
- ¼ Cup of shredded cheddar cheese

DIRECTIONS:

1. Preheat your oven to a temperature of about 400° F.
2. Microwave your cauliflower for about 5 minutes.
3. In the meantime; add the beef to a large skillet and sprinkle with the steak seasoning on top
4. Add in the cauliflower, the cream cheese and the shredded cheddar cheese.
5. Mix your ingredients very well; then pour the mixture into a baking dish
6. In a medium bowl; beat the eggs; then whisk in the cream and the butter
7. Pour over the beef mixture and top with the remaining quantity of cheese
8. Bake for about 30 minutes.
9. Serve and enjoy your dish!

NURITION

Kcal: 499.8 Fat: 40.1 Carbs: 5.5 Proteins: 29.2

INSTANT POT BEEF AND CAJUN RICE

Prep Time: 15 Minutes| Cooking Time: 15 Minutes| Servings: 3-4

INGREDIENTS

- 2 Tablespoons of oil
- 1 and ½ cups of fresh diced onion
- 1 Cup of diced bell peppers
- ½ Cup of diced celery
- 1 Pound of chopped beef
- 1 Tablespoon of salt-free Cajun seasoning
- 1 Cup of water
- 1 Teaspoon of salt
- 2 Bay leaves
- 1 Teaspoon of dried oregano
- 2 Teaspoons of hot sauce
- 1 Cup of rinsed and drained long-grain white rice

DIRECTIONS:

1. Turn on your Instant Pot by pressing the button "Sauté" and when it displays hot, add in the oil; then add in the chopped beef and stir for 4 minutes
2. Add in the bay leaf, the Cajun seasoning, the hot sauce, the salt and the rice; then stir for 3 minutes
3. Pour in the broth and lock the lid.
4. Make sure to seal the valve and cook on High pressure for about 5 minutes.
5. When the timer beeps, let the Instant Pot rest for about 10 minutes
6. Release the remaining pressure; then fluff the rice with a fork
7. Serve and enjoy your dish!

NURITION

Kcal: 461 Fat: 18 Carbs: 43 Proteins: 26

SEAFOOD AND FISH RECIPES

BAKED FLOUNDER

Prep Time: 8 Minutes| Cooking Time: 15 Minutes| Servings: 3

INGREDIENTS:

- The juice of 1 lemon or lime
- ½ Cup of extra virgin olive oil
- ½ Cup of unsalted melted coconut oil
- 1 Thinly sliced shallot
- 1 Thinly sliced garlic clove
- 1 Tablespoon of capers
- 1 Teaspoon of seasoned salt
- Teaspoon of ground black pepper
- 1 Teaspoon of ground cumin
- 1Teaspoon of garlic powder
- ½ Pounds of flounder
- 2 Trimmed green onions from the top; cut the onion lengthwise
- 1 Sliced lime or lemon
- ¾ Cup of chopped fresh dill

DIRECTIONS :

1. In a small bowl, mix altogether the olive oil with the melted coconut oil
2. Season with a little bit of the seasoned salt and add the shallots, the garlic and the capers.
3. In a separate bowl; mix the seasoned salt with the pepper, the cumin and the garlic powder.
4. Spice the fish fillets, each on both its sides.
5. Put the fish fillets into a greased large baking tray; then cover with the mixture of lime that you have already prepared.
6. Arrange the onion halves and the limes right on top
7. Bake your dish in the oven for about 15 minutes at a heat of about 375° F
8. Remove the fish from your oven and garnish it with toppings of your choice; but first don't forget to garnish with the fresh dill.
9. Serve and enjoy with a salad of your choice!

NURITION

Kcal: 142.1 Fat: 4 Carbs: 1.5 Proteins: 24.6

SPICY SCALLOPS WITH LEMON

Prep Time: 5 Minutes| Cooking Time: 5 Minutes| Servings: 2-3

INGREDIENTS

- ½ Pound of large scallops
- 1 Tablespoon of clarified ghee
- 1Grated garlic clove
- The zest of 1 lemon
- ¼ Cup of chopped Italian parsley
- ½ Teaspoon of sea salt
- ¼ Teaspoon of freshly ground peppercorn
- ¼ Teaspoon of red pepper flakes
- 1 pinch of sweet paprika
- 1 Teaspoon of extra virgin olive oil

DIRECTIONS :

1. Start by patting dry all of your scallops with a paper towel very well.
2. Heat a non-stick skillet over a medium heat
3. Put the scallops with a little bit of olive oil and sprinkle it with a little bit of sea salt, a little bit of cracked pepper, the red pepper flakes and with sweet paprika.
4. Toss the scallops to coat it and add a little bit of ghee to your hot skillet
5. Add in the scallops to the pan and sear it for about 3 to 5 minutes
6. Add the ghee to your skillet and the scallops; then stir in the garlic and remove the ingredients from the heat
7. Squeeze half of your lemon on top of the scallops.
8. Garnish with parsley and lemon zest
9. Serve and enjoy your dish!

NURITION Kcal: 306 Fat: 43 Carbs: 14.3 Proteins: 14

SALMON WITH DILL

Prep Time: 10 Minutes| Cooking Time: 2 Hours| Servings: 4

INGREDIENTS

- 1 to 2 Pounds of salmon
- 2 Minced garlic cloves
- 1 Handful of fresh dill
- 1 Sliced lemon
- 1 Pinch of salt
- 1 Pinch of pepper
- ½ Teaspoon of olive oil

DIRECTIONS :

1. Line a 4 quart slow cooker with a parchment paper.
2. Season the salmon with 1 pinch of salt, 1 pinch of pepper, the garlic, and the fresh dill.
3. Lay the salmon over the parchment paper
4. Top the salmon with the lemon slices and the oil
5. Cover your slow cooker with a lid and cook on HIGH for about 1 to 2 hours.
6. When the time is up; turn off your slow cooker
7. Serve and enjoy your salmon dish!

NURITION
Kcal: 199.1 Fat: 8.2 Carbs: 2 Proteins: 29.1

COCONUT CRUSTED SHRIMP

Prep Time: 10 Minutes| Cooking Time: 5 Minutes| Servings: 3

INGREDIENTS:

- 1 Pound of large peeled and deveined shrimps
- 1 Large egg
- ¼ Teaspoon of black pepper
- ¼ Teaspoon of salt
- 1 Cup of unsweetened shredded coconut
- Coconut oil for frying

DIRECTIONS :

1. In a medium shallow bowl, crack in the eggs and beat it with the salt and the black pepper; then set it aside
2. Put the shredded coconut into a large plate.
3. Dip each of the shrimps into the egg wash; then press each shrimp into the coconut
4. Now, pour the coconut oil into a large non-stick skillet over a medium heat
5. Fry your shrimps for about 3 to 4 minutes per batch
6. Serve the shrimp with your favourite sauce
7. Enjoy!

NURITION
Kcal: 309 Fat: 13.2 Carbs: 14.3 Proteins: 8.8

DUTCH OVEN SARDINES WITH HERBS

Prep Time: 10 Minutes| Cooking Time: 10 Minutes| Servings: 3

INGREDIENTS:

- 1 Pound of rinsed and cleaned fresh sardines, patted dry
- 1 Minced garlic clove
- 2 Teaspoons of French mustard
- 1 Tablespoon of lemon juice plus lemon for serving
- 1 Tablespoon of dry oregano
- ½ Teaspoon of paprika
- 1 Teaspoon of dry onion flakes
- ¼ Teaspoon of salt
- 1 Pinch of freshly ground pepper
- 3 Tablespoons of olive oil
- 2 Teaspoons of fresh parsley chopped

DIRECTIONS:

1. Preheat your oven at a temperature of about 430° F with the fan on.
2. In a large bowl; combine all the ingredients except for the fresh parsley and the sardines
3. Add the sardines to the same bowl and gently so that all your sardines are very well coated.
4. Grease a Dutch oven with a small quantity of cooking dish with a small quantity of olive oil; then place the sardines in one layer and drizzle any leftover dressing on top of the fish
5. Roast the fish for about 15 to 17 minutes or more if needed
6. Roast for 15-17 minutes a bit more
7. Remove the sardines from the Dutch oven and sprinkle fresh parsley on top; then squeeze a little quantity of lemon
8. Serve and enjoy your dish!

NURITION

Kcal: 339 Fat: 14 Carbs: 9.9 Proteins: 43

SPICY HALIBUT

Prep Time: 10 Minutes| Cooking Time: 10 Minutes| Servings: 2-3

INGREDIENTS:

- 2 Cups of packed spinach
- 2 Halibut fish meat
- The Juice of half a lemon
- 1 Pinch of salt
- 1 Pinch of pepper
- 1 Pinch of smoked paprika
- 1 sliced lemon
- ½ Sliced green onions
- 1 Deseeded and thinly sliced red chili
- 1 Cup of halved cherry tomatoes
- 2 tbsp of avocado oil

DIRECTIONS :

1. Place two squares of the same size of halibut fish over a flat surface
2. Divide the spinach between the squares
3. Place the halibut over a chopping board; then remove the membrane and the bone
4. You should have about 5 pieces all in all
5. Lay the first 2 pieces of halibut over each of the spinach piles; then squeeze the lemon over each part
6. Season with smoke paprika
7. Top with lemon slices
8. Top each fillet with the sliced green onions, the chili and the cherry tomatoes
9. Pour 1 tbsp of avocado oil over each fish portion
10. Tightly wrap the foil around the fish; then arrange the two in the flat pan
11. Leave to cook for 10 minutes
12. Remove when the fish turns into gold
13. Serve and enjoy your dinner!

NURITION

Kcal: 233.5 Fat: 6.9 Carbs: 7.9 Proteins: 30.5

COD FISH WITH TOMATO SAUCE

Prep Time: 10 Minutes| Cooking Time: 15 Minutes| Servings: 2

INGREDIENTS:

To make the Tomato Sauce:
- 2 Tablespoons of olive oil
- ½ Teaspoon of crushed red pepper flakes
- 2 Large, finely minced garlic cloves
- 1 Sliced pint of cherry tomatoes
- ¼ Cup of dry white wine
- ½ Cup of finely chopped fresh basil
- 2 Tablespoons of fresh lemon juice

- ½ Teaspoon of fresh lemon zest
- ½ Teaspoon of salt
- ¼ Teaspoon of fresh ground black pepper

To prepare the Cod:
- 2 Tablespoons of olive oil
- ½ Pound of fresh and cut cod
- 1 Pinch of salt and 1 pinch of pepper

DIRECTIONS :

1. Preheat your oven to about 375° F

To make the tomato sauce:

2. Heat the oil in a large pan over a medium heat
3. Add the crushed red pepper flakes and the garlic; then sauté the ingredients altogether for about 1 to 2 minutes
4. Add the tomatoes and cook the ingredients for about 13 minutes; but make sure to stir from time to time
5. Pour in the white wine and let simmer; then add the basil, the lemon juice, the lemon zest, the salt and the pepper and cook for about 2 minutes
6. Transfer your sauce to a medium bowl; then set it aside

To make the Cod:

7. Heat the oil in a large skillet and sauté it over a medium heat.
8. Season both the sides of the Cod with the salt and the pepper.
9. Put the cod into the oil and cook it for about 4 minutes
10. Flip the cod from time to time and bake it in the oven for about 5 minutes
11. Pour the wine over the tomato basil sauce and serve it.
12. Enjoy your dish!

NURITION

Kcal: 338.4 Fat: 26.7 Carbs: 9.5 Proteins: 11.2

BAKED TROUT

Prep Time: 10 Minutes| Cooking Time: 40 Minutes| Servings: 6

INGREDIENTS:
- 6 Trouts of about 20 cm each
- 12 Slices of Bacon
- 1 Teaspoon of ground Pepper
- The Bacon on the Trout

DIRECTIONS:
1. Start by filleting the trout.
2. Lay about three slices of bacon on the bottom of a Dutch oven
3. Put about half of a trout with the flesh-side-down, on each of the sliced.
4. Sprinkle 1 pinch of pepper lightly on top of upper sides of fish.
5. Arrange a second layer of bacon and the fish at right angles to the first.
6. Continue to arrange other layers of fish
7. Cover your Dutch oven and bury in coals
8. Cook for about 35 to 40 minutes
9. Serve your delicious dish with bacon and enjoy with each with half a fish.

NURITION
Kcal: 352 Fat: 4.6 Carbs: 18.9 Proteins: 45

DUTCH OVEN BAKED SALMON

Prep Time: 10 Minutes| Cooking Time: 11 Minutes| Servings: 4

INGREDIENTS:
- Extra virgin olive oil
- 2 Sliced shallots
- 1 Thinly sliced and rinsed leek; only the green part
- 2 Sliced carrots
- 1 Sliced fennel bulb
- 1 Pint of sliced grape tomatoes
- 2 Sliced medium zucchini
- 2 Sliced garlic cloves
- 1 Piece of 2 inches of ginger
- Tarragon; several thyme or basil sprigs
- 1 Cup of dry white wine
- 2 Cups of water
- 4 Skinned salmons, 6 ounces
- 1 Pinch of kosher salt
- 1 Pinch of freshly ground black pepper
- Fresh chopped fresh herbs
- A drizzle of oil

DIRECTIONS:
1. Heat a large Dutch oven coated with oil over a medium high heat
2. Then add the sweat shallots, the leek, the carrot and the fennel and stir for about 20 minutes
3. Add the tomatoes, the zucchini, the garlic, the ginger, the herbs, the wine, and the water and bring the mixture to a simmer.
4. Turn off the heat; then add the salmon to the Dutch oven and gently push it into the vegetables
5. Put the Dutch oven into your preheated oven and roast at a temperature of about 300°F, uncovered, for about 10 to 11 minutes.
6. Spoon the vegetables around the serving platter with some poaching liquid
7. Discard the ginger; then garnish with the fresh chopped herbs and oil

NURITION
Kcal: 255 Fat: 4.5 Carbs: 12 Proteins: 15

OVEN BAKED SHRIMP

Prep Time: 10 Minutes| Cooking Time: 10 Minutes| Servings: 3-4

INGREDIENTS:

- 1 and ¼ pounds of peeled wild shrimp
- 3 Minced garlic cloves garlic
- ½ Teaspoon of red pepper flakes
- 3 Tablespoons of lemon juice
- 3 Tablespoons of olive oil
- 2 Tablespoons of vegetable broth
- ¼ Cup of chopped tomatoes
- ¼ Teaspoon of salt
- ¼ Teaspoon of pepper
- 2 Tablespoons of fresh chopped parsley

DIRECTIONS:

1. Preheat your oven to about 375 degrees.
2. Place all the ingredients except for the parsley in a Cast iron Dutch oven
3. Bake for about 10 minutes
4. Remove from the oven and sprinkle the parsley on top
5. Serve and enjoy your dish!

NURITION

Kcal: 240 Fat: 10 Carbs: 8 Proteins: 28

FISH CURRY

Prep Time: 10 Minutes| Cooking Time: 5 Hours| Servings: 4

INGREDIENTS

- 1 Pound of Bigeye Jack
- 2 Cups of Coconut Milk
- 2 Diced tomatoes
- 4 Pieces of thinly sliced Jalapeno Peppers
- 1 Piece of thinly sliced Shallot
- 1 Crushed garlic Bulb
- 1 Piece of 2-inch thinly sliced ginger
- 2 Cups of chopped okra
- 1 Piece of chopped carrot
- 1 Teaspoon of Fenugreek Seeds
- 1 Stick of cinnamon
- 1 Teaspoon of Coriander Seeds
- 3 to 4 Pieces of Star Anise
- ½ Teaspoon of Cumin Seeds
- ½ Teaspoon of Mustard Seeds
- 2 Pieces of Bay Leaf
- 3 Tablespoons of Curry Powder

DIRECTIONS :

1. Gut the fish and scale it; then heat the oil in a wok and toast the cinnamon, the fenugreek, the coriander seeds, the star anise, the cumin seeds and the mustard seeds for about 1 to 2 minutes
2. Add the shallots, the garlic, the ginger, the jalapenos, and the tomatoes and sauté for about 1 minute.
3. Add the curry powder and cook for about 1 additional minute
4. Transfer your mixture to your slow cooker and pour in the coconut milk
5. Cover the slow cooker with its lid and cook on Low for about 4 hours on Low
6. When the time is up; turn off your slow cooker and turn the heat to high
7. Add the fish and cook for about 1 additional hour
8. Season with 1 pinch of salt and pepper
9. Serve and enjoy the fish dish!

NURITION

Kcal: 364 Fat: 21.3 Carbs: 8 Proteins: 28

LEGUMES

ARTICHOKE DIP

Prep Time 10 Minutes | Cooking Time:10 Minutes | Servings 4

INGREDIENTS:
- 1 Pound of artichoke leaves
- 2 cups of chickpeas
- 55 cl of olive oil
- 15 ml lemon juice
- 1 tsp of fresh mint, chopped

DIRECTIONS:
1. Bring a large pot of water to a boil, and then add the artichoke leaves. Cook for about 1 hour, stirring occasionally.
2. Drain; put the leaves in a food processor or a blender
3. Put the rest of the ingredients (half the mint only) in a blender and blend until you get a smooth consistency. Serve with the rest of the mint.
4. Serve and enjoy your dish!

NUTRITION
KCAL100g PRO 4g CARB 6g FAT 5g

FRUIT SKEWERS

Prep Time 10 Minutes | Cooking Time: 0Minutes | Servings 2-4

INGREDIENTS:
- ½ Pound of watermelon
- ½ green Melon
- ½ Melon
- 2 tablespoons of fresh mint
- 2 tablespoons of basil
- 45 ml of lemon juice
- 3 tablespoons of agave syrup

DIRECTIONS:
1. Start by making balls of the 2 melons and the watermelon with a small spoon.
2. Assemble the skewers alternating the melons and watermelon with a basil leaf.
3. Mix all together the mint, the basil, the lemon juice and the agave syrup
4. Drizzle with the vinaigrette on the skewers
5. Serve and enjoy your sumptuous fruit skewers!

NUTRITION
KCAL100g PRO 4g CARB 6g FAT 5g

BROCCOLI PICKLES

Prep Time 10 Minutes | Cooking Time: 0 Minutes | Servings 4

INGREDIENTS:

- ½ Pound of broccoli stalks, cut into rings
- 25 cl of white vinegar
- 25 cl of water
- 2 tablespoon of coarse salt
- 1 garlic clove, peeled
- 1 bay leaf

DIRECTIONS:

1. Sterilize a jar and then dry it.
2. Blanch the broccoli slices for 2 minutes. Immerse them in cold water. Put them in the jar.
3. In a saucepan, boil the vinegar with the salt water, the garlic and the bay leaf. Pour over the broccoli.
4. Close very well and seal the container; then keep for about 2 weeks before tasting.
5. Enjoy your pickles !

NUTRITION
KCAL240g PRO 0g CARB 17g FAT 0g

VEGETABLE PIE

Prep Time 15 Minutes | Cooking Time: 35 Minutes | Servings 6

INGREDIENTS:

- ½ Pound of turnip
- 1 beet
- ½ pound of cauliflower
- 2 red onion, thinly sliced
- 2 garlic cloves, minced
- 2 tablespoons of Thyme
- 2 tablespoons of rosemary
- 2 tablespoons of olive oil
- ½ pound of chard, chopped
- 2 ½ cups of cooked chickpeas, rinsed and drained
- 1 puff pastry

DIRECTIONS:

1. Preheat the oven to 400 ° F; cut the turnips, beets and cauliflower into 2 cm pieces.
2. Put them in a salad bowl with the onion, garlic, thyme, rosemary, olive oil, salt and pepper and mix well. Place them on the oven rack covered with baking paper and bake for 20 minutes until tender. Let cool. Add the chard and chickpeas, mix.
3. Preheat the oven to 400°F again if it has cooled too much. Place the dough in the middle of an oiled mold; then place the vegetables.
4. Fold the dough over the vegetables, pressing down to seal.
5. Bake for about 30 to 35 minutes.

NUTRITION
KCAL194g PRO 5g CARB 32g FAT 4g

ZUCCHINI SKEWERS

Prep Time 10 Minutes | Cooking Time: 10 Minutes | Servings 3

INGREDIENTS:

- 6 mini zucchinis; cut into 5cm pieces
- For the Marinade
- 60 ml of olive oil
- 1 lemon, the zest of juice
- 1 tsp of pepper
- 1 tablespoon of agave syrup
- 1 tablespoon of oregano

DIRECTIONS:

1. Place the zucchini in a deep dish. Prepare the marinade by mixing all the ingredients.
2. Pour the marinade over the zucchini and let marinate for at least 4 hours.
3. Place the zucchini pieces on the skewers and grill on the barbecue for a few minutes
4. Serve with the marinade to soak them.
5. Enjoy your zucchini skewers

NUTRITION

KCAL172 PRO 2g CARB 9g FAT 5g

GRILLED EGGPLANTS

Prep Time 10 Minutes | Cooking Time: 15 Minutes | Servings 5

INGREDIENTS:

- 2 eggplants
- 2 teaspoons of salt
- 1/2 cup extra virgin olive oil
- 3 crushed garlic cloves
- 2 tablespoons of chopped fresh parsley
- 2 tablespoons of chopped fresh oregano
- 1/2 tsp of pepper
- 1/4 teaspoon of salt

DIRECTIONS:

1. Start by cutting the eggplant into 1/4-inch-thick slices and generously salt each slice. Let them sit for about 15 minutes so that the salt can remove the moisture and bitterness. Wipe down each of the slices with a paper towel to remove salt and moisture.
2. Preheat the barbecue to medium heat
3. In a large dish, combine all together the olive oil, the garlic, parsley, the oregano, the salt and the pepper. Place each of the slices of the eggplants in the dish, turning them over to make sure both the sides are very well coated with oil.
4. Grill for about 6 minutes per side until golden brown with grill marks. If the eggplant slices get dry and sticky to the grill, brush them with more oil.
5. Once the eggplant is tender and cooked
6. Remove from the grill and return to the oil, herb and garlic mixture in the pan. Turn once so that both sides are coated before transferring to a serving dish. Place excess herbs and garlic on top before serving. Eggplant is best enjoyed hot or at room temperature and can be kept for up to 4 days in the refrigerator.
7. Serve and enjoy your grilled eggplants!

NUTRITION

KCAL 229 PRO 6g CARB 25g FAT 10g

ROASTED VEGETABLES

Prep Time 15 Minutes | Cooking Time: 60 Minutes | Servings 3-4

INGREDIENTS:

- 1Pound of turnips
- 1 Pound of carrots
- 3 zucchini
- 2 onions
- 3 cloves of garlic
- 2 tablespoons of duck fat (or olive oil)
- thyme and bay leaf
- Salt and pepper

DIRECTIONS:

1. Peel the vegetables.
2. Cut the onions and turnips into large cubes.
3. Cut the carrots into sticks.
4. Cut the zucchini into large cubes.
5. Blanch the carrots for 3 minutes in simmering water.
6. Do the same with the turnips.
7. Drain; then heat the fat and brown the onions in a roasting pan or sauté pan that can be oven-safe.
8. Add the crushed garlic, thyme and bay leaf.
9. Add the carrot sticks and color them without damaging them.
10. Then add the turnips.
11. Mix gently while browning over moderate heat then add the zucchini.
12. Season and place in the oven at 400°F for a quarter of an hour if you like vegetables that are still a little firm.
13. Stir during the cooking process
14. Serve and enjoy your roasted vegetables!

NUTRITION

KCAL90 PRO g CARB 17g FAT 2g

VEGETABLE TABBOULEH

Prep Time 10 Minutes | Cooking Time: 15 Minutes | Servings 4

INGREDIENTS:

- 1 Pound of Couscous semolina medium grain
- 3 Tomatoes
- 1/2 Cucumber
- 3 small white onions
- 1 lemon
- 3 tablespoons of olive oil
- 3 sprigs of Mint
- 3 sprigs of flat parsley
- 1 pinch of salt and pepper

DIRECTIONS:

1. Start this homemade oriental tabbouleh recipe by pouring the semolina into a large bowl. Salt, add the same volume of boiling water and let swell for 15 minutes. Then separate the grains with a fork.
2. Wash, seed the tomatoes; cut them into very small cubes. Peel, seed and cut the cucumber into small cubes. Peel and slice the onions. Squeeze the juice from the lemon. Wash, thin out and finely chop the herbs.
3. Mix the semolina with all the vegetables. Drizzle with the olive oil and the lemon juice
4. Add in the mint and the parsley leaves; then mix and adjust the seasoning.
5. Place in the fridge covered with cling film for 1 hour before eating.
6. Serve and enjoy your tabbouleh!

NUTRITION

KCAL286 PRO 6.5g CARB 37g FAT 14.5g

MUSHROOM STUFFED SQUASH

Prep Time 15 Minutes | Cooking Time: 20 Minutes | Servings 5

INGREDIENTS:

- 2 small squashes
- ½ Pound of button mushrooms
- 1 cup of dried porcini mushrooms
- 1 medium onion
- 2 cloves of garlic
- 1 cup of risotto rice
- 30 cl of vegetable broth
- 10 cl of dry white wine
- 2 tablespoons of grated Parmesan
- ½ bunch of chives
- 1 Tablespoons of olive oil
- 1 pinch of salt and 1 pinch of pepper

DIRECTIONS:

1. Soak the dried porcini mushrooms in 20 cl of water.
2. Slice them. Cut the squash in half.
3. Seed them, Place them on a baking sheet covered with parchment paper.
4. Add salt and pepper; then drizzle with a drizzle of oil.
5. Place for 30 minutes in the oven preheated to 400°F
6. Clean and slice the button mushrooms. Brown them in a pan with 1 tbsp of oil
7. Season with salt and pepper; then peel and mince the onion, chop the garlic.
8. Sauté them in a drizzle of oil
9. Add the rice and stir for a few minutes
10. Pour in the white wine, then the broth little by little
11. Season with salt and pepper.
12. Cook for about 15 to 20 minutes until the liquid has completely evaporated.
13. Add the flesh of the squash, the button mushrooms and the porcini mushrooms.
14. Stir in the Parmesan; mix for a few minutes. Divide the mixture among the squash halves.
15. Sprinkle with chopped chives.
16. Serve and enjoy your stuffed squash!

NUTRITION

KCAL145 PRO 6g CARB 15.38g FAT 7g

CAULIFLOWER CURRY

Prep Time 10 Minutes | Cooking Time: 23 Minutes | Servings 4

INGREDIENTS:

- 2 Tablespoons of vegetable oil
- 1 Small diced onion
- 1 Seeded and diced jalapeño
- 1 Tablespoon of grated fresh ginger
- ¼ Cup of red curry paste
- 1 Can of coconut milk
- 1 Can of diced tomatoes
- 1 Head of cauliflower
- 1 and ½ teaspoons of Kosher salt
- 1 Pinch of fresh ground black pepper

DIRECTIONS:

1. In a large saucepan, heat your oil over a medium heat.
2. Stir in the onion and the jalapeño; then cook the mixture until it becomes tender for 3 minutes
3. Stir in the ginger and cook your ingredients; stir from time to time
4. Add the curry paste and cook it for about 1 minute
5. Toss in the cauliflower florets with ½ cup of water.
6. Season your curry with 1 pinch of salt and 1 pinch of pepper.
7. Bring the ingredients to a boil and lower the heat and let it simmer until for 15 minutes
8. Serve and enjoy your cauliflower curry!

NUTRITION

KCAL123.8 PRO 4.3g CARB 18.9g FAT 4.6g

SNACK AND APPETIZERS

SPICY NACHOS IN SKILLET

Prep Time 10 Minutes | Cooking Time: 30 Minutes | Servings 5

INGREDIENTS:
- 2 tablespoons of olive oil
- 2 garlic cloves, minced
- 1 shallot, minced
- 1 1/2 to 2 cups of fresh mushrooms
- 1 tablespoon of cornstarch
- ¼ cup of water
- 2 Pounds of zucchini, cut into thin rings
- 1 pinch of salt and pepper

DIRECTIONS:
1. Heat the olive oil in a pan over medium heat, then sauté the garlic and shallot for 4 minutes. Clean the chanterelles and cut them in 4 lengthwise.
2. Cook for 10 minutes in the butter, then add the cornstarch and water and stir well.
3. Add the zucchini, season with salt and pepper and cook until the zucchini is tender, about 20 minutes.
4. Serve and enjoy your dish!

NUTRITION
KCAL: 205 FAT: 8.4g CARB: 11.6g PRO: 5.8g

POTATO PANCAKES

Prep Time 10 Minutes | Cooking Time: 30 Minutes | Servings 6

INGREDIENTS:
- 7 potatoes
- 2 eggs
- 1 red onion
- 1 branch parsley
- 1 pinch of salt
- 1 pinch pepper
- 1 c. olive oil

DIRECTIONS:
1. Peel and wash the potatoes; then grate them finely and put them in a salad bowl
2. Peel and roughly chop the onion. Mix it finely with the parsley
3. In the bowl containing the grated potatoes, add the eggs, the onion / parsley mixture, salt and pepper
4. Mix by hand; then heat a pan with olive oil
5. Make potato pancakes about 10 cm in diameter and brown the first side for 3 minutes
6. Potato pancakes
7. Turn the patties over and brown the second side for 3 minutes too
8. Do the same until all the mixture is used up
9. Serve and enjoy your snack hot!

NUTRITION
KCAL170PRO 2.6g CARB 26g FAT 5g

GRILLED CAULIFLOWER

Prep Time 10 Minutes | Cooking Time: 15 Minutes | Servings 4

INGREDIENTS:

- 1 head of cauliflower, cut into large pieces
- 3 tablespoons of olive oil
- 1 teaspoon of coarse salt
- 1 and ½ teaspoons of crushed black pepper

DIRECTIONS:

1. Preheat the barbecue to medium heat and lightly oil the grill.
2. In a bowl, combine the cauliflower with the oil
3. Season with the salt and the pepper
4. Cook the cauliflower pieces on the hot grill for about 10-15 minutes in total, making sure to turn every 2 minutes
5. Serve and enjoy your grilled cauliflower!

NUTRITION

KCA: 88g PRO 2g CARB 8g FAT 3g

COOKED COCO BEANS

Prep Time 10 Minutes | Cooking Time: 35Minutes | Servings 4

INGREDIENTS:

- 2 Pounds of fresh Paimpol coconut beans
- 2 bay leaves
- 1 sprig of thyme
- 1 clove of garlic
- A few sprigs of fresh parsley
- Olive oil
- 1 Pinch of Salt
- 1 Pinch of ground Pepper

DIRECTIONS:

1. Shell the beans and rinse them.
2. Place the beans in a large saucepan with the thyme, the peeled, and halved garlic clove, and the bay leaf
3. Cover with plenty of water..
4. Let simmer for about for 35 minutes.
5. Drain the beans and mix them with the tomato sauce in a saucepan. Season with salt and pepper and reheat over low heat for about ten minutes, stirring frequently.
6. Serve and enjoy your dish!

NUTRITION

KCAL160 PRO 4g CARB 12g FAT 8g

CARAMELIZED CARROTS

Prep Time 10 Minutes | Cooking Time: 20 Minutes | Servings 6

INGREDIENTS:
- 2 Pounds of carrots
- 1 Cup of vegan butter
- 1 tablespoon of powdered sugar
- 2 tablespoon of chopped parsley
- 1 Pinch of salt
- 1 Pinch of pepper

PREPARATION:
1. To easily make your carrots, start by preparing the vegetables. To do this, quickly scrape the carrots with a peeler or a vegetable peeler, or even with a knife.
2. Wash them thoroughly under a stream of cold water; then cut them into large slices and set them aside.
3. In a large Dutch oven, heat the butter and powdered sugar. Mix well until you obtain light foam.
4. Be careful not to burn the butter and not to form a caramel with the sugar.
5. To make the caramelized carrots; then add the carrot slices and brown them for a few minutes, stirring with a wooden spoon or spatula. Then cover them with water and season to taste with salt and pepper.
6. Cook, half covered and over a medium heat, until the water has evaporated (about 20 min) without mixing. Then add the parsley that you have previously washed and finely chopped, mix and check the cooking with a knife blade. When the carrots are cooked, they should be very tender.
7. Continue cooking over low heat if necessary, stirring regularly so that the carrots do not stick or adding a little water if necessary. Turn off the heat.
8. Serve and enjoy your caramelized carrots!

NUTRITION
KCAL133.2 PRO 1.6g CARB 11.9g FAT 9.6g

PLANT-BASED FRITATTA

Prep Time 15 Minutes | Cooking Time: 60 Minutes | Servings 5

INGREDIENTS:
- ½ eggplant cut into 2cm cubes
- 1 zucchini, cut into 2cm cubes
- ½ yellow onion, minced
- ½ pound of cherry tomatoes
- 1 tablespoon of basil
- ½ tablespoon of oregano
- 30 ml olive oil
- 1 garlic clove, chopped
- 5 large eggs
- 20 ml milk
- ½ cup of grated Parmesan

DIRECTIONS:
1. Preheat your oven to 400°F. Place the eggplant, zucchini, onion and cherry tomatoes in a salad bowl. Sprinkle with basil, oregano, 1 tbsp of olive oil, salt and pepper. Mix the vegetables then place them on the baking sheet covered with baking paper. Roast the vegetables for 40 minutes, stirring regularly.
2. When the vegetables are almost roasted, add the remaining olive oil to an ovenproof pan. Place the pan over medium heat and add the garlic. Sauté for 1-2 minutes, add the grilled vegetables, mix.
3. Whisk the eggs and milk in a bowl, and then pour them over the vegetables in the pan. Sprinkle with Parmesan and put in the oven for about 10 to 15 minutes.
4. Serve and enjoy your frittata!

NUTRITION
KCAL441g PRO 10g CARB 48g FAT 26g

VEGGIE MAKI SUSHI

Prep Time 20 Minutes | Cooking Time: 30 Minutes | Servings 6

INGREDIENTS:

- ½ Pound of round white rice
- 1 tablespoon of sugar
- 1 tablespoon of rice vinegar
- 250 ml of water
- The garnish:
- ½ of a cucumber
- ½ pound of carrots
- 2 avocados
- 3 nori seaweed sheets
- For the sauce
- 2 wasabi nuts
- 10 cl soy sauce
- 1 tablespoons of ginger

DIRECTIONS:

1. Wash the rice grains 4 times with cold water. Drain and let stand 25 minutes.
2. In a bowl, combine the sugar, rice vinegar and a little salt until combined; reserve
3. Pour the rice and the indicated amount of water into the pot, cover. Start cooking over a medium heat
4. When it comes to a boil, reduce the heat; stir the rice a little with a spatula. Then, still covered, continue cooking over low heat for 10-12 minutes. Remove the pan from the heat and let stand for 10 minutes.
5. Pour the rice into a salad bowl. Carefully separate the rice grains with a spatula, while gradually basting them with the rice vinegar mixture. Let cool before making the maki.
6. Remove the skin from the avocado. Cut it into thin sticks. Wash, empty and peel the cucumber and carrots and cut them into thin sticks.
7. Cut the seaweed leaves in half lengthwise.
8. Place the nori half sheet flat on the makisu (bamboo mat), lengthwise, shiny side facing you.
9. Dip your fingers in the bowl of water to catch the rice, so that it does not stick to your fingers. Take about 1 cup of rice then spread it evenly over the nori sheet.
10. Place a small dab of wasabi in the center of the rice and spread it evenly.
11. Line one or more strips of cucumber, carrots and avocado in the center of the layer of rice, over the wasabi
12. Roll the maki. Cut each of the 6 rolls obtained in 6.
13. Serve with ginger, wasabi and soy sauce.

NUTRITION
KCAL: 193 FAT: 6g CARB: 30g PRO: 6g

ROASTED GREEN BEANS

Prep Time: 5 Minutes| Cooking Time: 25 Minutes| Servings: 3

INGREDIENTS

- 2 Cups of sliced fresh mushrooms
- 2 Cups of fresh green beans
- ¼ Cup of olive oil
- 2 Teaspoons of minced garlic
- 1 Teaspoon of freshly ground sea salt
- 1 Teaspoon of freshly ground pepper

DIRECTIONS:

1. Preheat your oven to a temperature of about 400°F.
2. Wash your mushrooms; then slice it
3. Slice the green beans; then combine it with the oil, the garlic, the salt and the pepper in a separate bowl
4. Pour the oil over the mushrooms; then add the green bean and stir very well until your vegetables are very well coated
5. Place your veggies over a baking sheet; then bake it for about 20 to 25 minutes
6. Remove the veggies from the oven; then serve and enjoy your dish!

NURITION
Kcal: 100.1 Fat: 8.1 Carbs: 8 Proteins: 2.2

SAVORY RYE WITH VINAIGRAITTE

Prep Time 10 Minutes | Cooking Time: 40 Minutes | Servings 3-4

INGREDIENTS:

- ½ Pound of rye
- 2 avocado, diced
- 1 cup of dried plums, diced
- 3 tbsp of fresh mint
- 1 cup of roughly chopped pistachios

For the Vinaigrette:

- 1 tbsp of maple syrup
- 45 ml of olive oil
- 30 ml of lime juice

DIRECTIONS:

1. The day before, put the rye to soak in a bowl of cold water, placed in the refrigerator. The same day, cook the rye for about 40 minutes in boiling water.
2. Whisk the dressing ingredients together with a little salt.
3. Place the rye, apricots, avocado, mint and pistachios in a bowl
4. Drizzle with the vinaigrette, mix gently
5. Serve and enjoy your dish!

NUTRITION

KCAL223 PRO 10g CARB 48g FAT 26g

RICE GRATIN

Prep Time 20 Minutes | Cooking Time: 70 Minutes | Servings 5

INGREDIENTS:

- ½ Pound of rice
- 30 ml of olive oil
- 2 zucchini, sliced
- 3 tomatoes, sliced
- 1 onion, minced

- 1 garlic clove, crushed
- 2 eggs, whipped
- 1 cup of grated parmesan cheese
- 1 tablespoon of Thyme
- ½ cup of nuts

DIRECTIONS:

1. Preheat your oven to a temperature of about 420 ° F while you prepare the vegetables.
2. Put the zucchini in a salad bowl, sprinkle with half the olive oil, salt and pepper. Do the same with the tomatoes. Place the zucchini on the baking sheet covered with baking paper (leave room for the tomatoes). Bake for about 20 minutes.
3. After 10 minutes, add in the tomatoes.
4. In the meantime; cook the rice according to the directions of the package
5. Heat the oil in a pan, add the onion, garlic, salt and cook for 10 to 15 minutes, over low heat
6. Toast the pine nuts dry pine in a frying pan
7. In a salad bowl, mix the cooked rice, onion, eggs, thyme and half of the cheese, salt and pepper.
8. Grease a baking dish; then add in the rice mixture, then the zucchini, pine nuts, tomatoes and finish with the rest quantity of the cheese. Bake for about 15 to 20 minutes.
9. Serve and enjoy your appetizer!

NUTRITION

KCAL340g PRO 11g CARB 42g FAT 12g

VEGETABLE ZUCCHINI SUN PIE

Prep Time 10 Minutes | Cooking Time: 30 Minutes | Servings 4

INGREDIENTS:

- 30 ml olive oil
- 1 yellow onion, thinly sliced
- 1 garlic clove, minced
- 2 Tablespoons of tomato paste
- 1 eggplant, cut into slices of 1 inch each
- 1 zucchini
- 2 sprig of thyme
- 1 sprig of rosemary
- 1 tablespoon of agave syrup
- 1 puff pastry

DIRECTIONS:

1. Heat half the olive oil in a sauté pan. Add the onion, garlic, cook for 1 minute, add the tomato puree, half the thyme and the rosemary, season with salt and pepper, wet to the height, bring to a boil and cook until the sauce reduces a little . Reserve.
2. Heat the rest of the olive oil in a pan and cook the eggplants and zucchini in it until they are barely cooked.
3. Preheat the oven to 360° F.
4. Put the agave syrup at the bottom of a pie dish with the rest of the thyme and crumbled rosemary, salt and pepper. Arrange the eggplants and zucchini, overlapping them. Add the onion mixture on top. Cover with the dough, prick it and bake for 30 minutes.
5. Let cool a little bit
6. Serve and enjoy your appetizer!

NUTRITION

KCAL449g PRO 8g CARB 48g FAT 30g

MIXED ROASTED NUTS

Prep Time: 6 Minutes| Cooking Time: 20 Minutes| Servings: 2

INGREDIENTS:

- 2 Cups of mixed nuts; walnut, almonds and cashews
- 1 Tablespoon of garlic infused in olive oil
- 1 Pinch of smoked sea salt to taste
- 1 Pinch of smoked sweet paprika
- 1 Pinch of smoked hot paprika

DIRECTIONS :

1. Preheat your oven to about 325° F.
2. Combine the nuts into a large bowl and drizzle with the olive oil until your ingredients are very-well coated.
3. Combine the salt and the spices into a small bowl.
4. Sprinkle the spices over the nuts and stir very well until your nuts are combined
5. Spread the nuts into one layer over a baking sheet; then bake in the oven for about 20 minutes
6. Serve and enjoy!

NURITION

Kcal: 168 Fat: 15 Carbs: 7.2 Proteins: 4.9

ROASTED VEGGIES

Prep Time: 6 Minutes| Cooking Time: 30 Minutes| Servings: 3

INGREDIENTS

- 1 Pound of cleaned cremini mushrooms
- 2 Cups of diced cauliflower
- 2 Cups of cocktail tomatoes
- 12 Peeled garlic cloves
- 2 Tablespoons of olive oil
- 1 Tablespoon of Italian seasoning
- 1 Pinch of salt
- 1 Pinch of black pepper
- 1 Tablespoon of fresh, chopped parsley

DIRECTIONS:

1. Preheat your oven to a temperature of about 400° F
2. Place the mushrooms and the veggies into a medium bowl
3. Drizzle the veggies with a little bit of olive
4. Add the Italian seasoning, the salt, the pepper; then toss your ingredients very well
5. Place your veggies over a baking sheet; then place it in your preheated oven
6. Bake your veggies for about 20 to 30 minutes
7. Garnish your veggies with finely minced fresh parsley
8. Serve and enjoy your roasted veggies!

NURITION

Kcal: 122.2 Fat: 6.1 Carbs: 14 Proteins: 6

ROASTED OKRA

Prep Time: 5 Minutes| Cooking Time: 15 Minutes| Servings: 4

INGREDIENTS

- 12 Oz of thawed frozen baby okra
- 3 Tablespoons fat of avocado oil
- ½ Teaspoon of cumin seeds
- 1 Diced onion
- 1 Minced Serrano pepper
- 2 Minced garlic cloves
- ½ Inch of minced ginger
- ¼ Teaspoon of turmeric
- ¼ Teaspoon of salt

DIRECTIONS:

1. Start by rinsing the okra; then slice it into thin rounds
2. Spread the okra pieces over a paper towel and let dry; then prepare the remaining ingredients
3. The okra must be dry; then add in the cumin seeds and sauté it for about 1 minute
4. Add the Serrano pepper and the onions; then sauté for about 10 minutes
5. Add the ginger and the spices; then mix very well
6. Reduce the heat; then add 1 tablespoon of olive oil
7. Sauté your ingredients for about 10 minutes
8. Add the ginger and the garlic
9. Add the spices; then lower the heat and add 1 tablespoon of avocado oil and add the okra
10. Fry the okra for about 10 to 12 minutes
11. Serve and enjoy your okra!

NURITION

Kcal: 102 Fat: 4.1 Carbs: 15 Proteins: 5.2

ROASTED BRUSSELS SPROUTS

Prep Time: 10 Minutes| Cooking Time: 15 Minutes| Servings: 4-5

INGREDIENTS

- 1 Pound of Brussels sprouts
- 2 Tablespoons of avocado oil
- ½ Teaspoon of sea salt
- ½ Teaspoon of pepper
- 1 Cup of Coconut Cream
- ½ Teaspoon of Nutmeg
- 1 Tablespoons of Lemon Juice
- ⅓ Cup of Pomegranate Seeds

DIRECTIONS:

1. Cut the end of the Brussels sprouts; then remove and discard the icky outer leaves of your Brussels sprouts.
2. Now, cut the Brussels sprouts into halves
3. Heat the oil in a pan over a medium high heat
4. Add the Brussels sprouts; then add 1 pinch of salt and 1 pinch of pepper
5. Cook the Brussels sprouts and stir from time to time for about 2 to 3 minutes
6. Decrease the heat; then add the coconut cream, the nutmeg and the lemon juice; stir very well and cover your pan.
7. Check the Brussels sprouts after about 15 minutes
8. Serve your side dish and top it with pomegranate seeds
9. Enjoy your side dish!

NURITION

Kcal: 153 Fat: 7.4 Carbs: 13 Proteins: 4.3

MASHED CAULIFLOWER

Prep Time: 10 Minutes| Cooking Time: 10 Minutes| Servings: 3

INGREDIENTS

- 1 Medium head of trimmed and chopped cauliflower
- 3 Garlic cloves
- 1 Tablespoon of extra virgin olive oil
- ½ Teaspoon of salt
- 1/8 Teaspoon of freshly ground black pepper
- To make the garnish:
- 1 Tablespoon of extra virgin olive oil
- 1 Pinch of salt
- 1 Pinch of freshly ground black pepper

DIRECTIONS:

1. Place a large and deep saucepan over a medium high heat
2. Add the garlic and the cauliflower; then let cook for about 9 to 10 minutes Let your ingredients, drain; then set it aside for about 2 minutes
3. Place the cauliflower into a food processor; then add the salt, the pepper and the olive oil
4. Garnish your lashed cauliflower with finely chopped fresh thyme, salt and pepper
5. Drizzle with a little bit of oil
6. Serve and enjoy your mashed cauliflower!

NURITION

Kcal: 142.1 Fat: 10.38 Carbs: 8.50 Proteins: 4.80

BAKED SUNFLOWER SEEDS

Prep Time: 5 Minutes| Cooking Time: 10 Minutes| Servings: 2

INGREDIENTS

- 1 Cup of sunflower seeds
- 2 Teaspoon of olive oil
- 1 Tablespoon of cayenne pepper
- ½ Teaspoon of sea salt

DIRECTIONS:

1. Place the sunflower seeds into a pot or pan over a medium heat.
2. Stir the sunflower seeds for about 3 to 5 minutes or until the seeds start making a crackling sound
3. Remove the sunflower seeds from the heat
4. Stir in the oil and the cayenne pepper
5. Season the sunflower seeds with sea salt
6. Let cool; then serve it and enjoy its incredibly delicious taste!

NURITION

Kcal: 132 Fat: 6.2 Carbs: 14 Proteins: 4.3

SWEET POTATO FINGERS

Prep Time: 5 Minutes| Cooking Time: 10 Minutes| Servings: 3

INGREDIENTS

- 2 Large peeled and cubed sweet potatoes
- ¼ Medium, finely diced medium onion
- 2 Tablespoons of all purpose flour
- 1 Teaspoon of garlic powder
- 1 Teaspoon of chili powder
- ½ Teaspoon of salt
- ¼ Teaspoon of freshly ground pepper
- ½ Cup of oil

DIRECTIONS:

1. Place a large and deep saucepan filled with water over a medium heat and let it boil
2. Add in the sweet potatoes; then let cook for about 5 minutes
3. Let the potatoes; drain and rinse it with cold water
4. Remove any excess of water
5. Put the sweet potatoes and the onion in a food processor; then pulse it into small pieces
6. Transfer the potatoes into a large bowl; then add the coconut flour; the chili powder, the salt and the pepper; stir very well
7. With your hands; make small cylinders; then place the potatoes aside to fry it
8. Place a large non-stick skillet over a medium high heat; then pour the oil in it
9. When the oil gets hot; add the mixture of the potatoes to the skillet; then fry it in 1 or more batches
10. Cook each batch of potatoes for about 2 to 3 minutes or until it becomes crispy
11. Place the potatoes over a plate lined with a paper towel
12. Repeat the same process with the remaining quantity of potato mixture
13. Serve and enjoy your dish!

NURITION

Kcal: 119 Fat: 5.2 Carbs: 16 Proteins: 5

ROASTED ALMONDS WITH SHREDDED COCONUT

Prep Time: 5 Minutes| Cooking Time: 10 Minutes| Servings: 3

INGREDIENTS:
- 1 Cup of shredded sweetened coconut
- 2 Cups of raw whole almonds
-

- 2   Tablespoons   of   honey

DIRECTIONS:
1. Start by placing the coconut into a large frying pan over a low heat
2. Stir your ingredients very well together until the coconut start to get a golden color
3. Remove the coconut from the pan; then transfer it to a food processor; then pulse it until you get small shreds; then set it aside
4. Beware of burning the coconut because it gets a bad odor when you do
5. Preheat your oven to a temperature of about 350°F.
6. Put the almonds over a cookie sheet; then line the sheet with parchment paper Bake the almonds for about 6 minutes
7. While your almonds are being toasted; then place the honey into a large bowl
8. When your almonds are perfectly cooked; remove it from the oven; then transfer it to a heat-proof bowl
9. Coat the almonds with the raw honey; then stir
10. Place the almonds into 1 single layer and let it dry for about 50 minutes
11. Serve and enjoy your almond snack!
12. You can also store the almonds in a container for about 1 week

NURITION
Kcal: 159.6 Fat: 14.1 Carbs: 7.1 Proteins: 6.3

BAKED PLANTAINS

Prep Time: 5 Minutes| Cooking Time: 20 Minutes| Servings: 3

INGREDIENTS
- 1 to 2 green plantains
- 1 Teaspoon of extra olive oil

- ½ Teaspoon of sea salt

DIRECTIONS:
1. Preheat your oven to a temperature of about 350° F
2. Line a baking sheet with a parchment paper
3. Cut the ends of the plantains
4. Score the plantain in a lengthwise way; then peel your plantain
5. Cut the plantain into slices; then toss the slices of the plantain with the oil
6. Lay the plantain over a baking sheet; then sprinkle it with salt
7. Bake your ingredient for about 19 minutes
8. Remove the plantains from the oven; then serve and enjoy your delicious snack!

NURITION
Kcal: 137.1 Fat: 2.36 Carbs: 13 Proteins: 2

BAKED PUMPKIN SEEDS

Prep Time: 5 Minutes| Cooking Time: 18 Minutes| Servings: 2

INGREDIENTS

- 2 Cups of pumpkin seeds
- 1 Teaspoon of vanilla extract
- 2 Teaspoons of maple syrup
- 2 Teaspoons of coconut sugar
- Boiled water

DIRECTIONS:

1. Preheat your oven to a temperature of about 290° F
2. In a large or medium bowl, combine altogether the coconut sugar, the honey and the vanilla; then stir altogether very well in order to create a paste
3. Add a drop of boiled water in order to create a kind of runny syrup
4. Place in the pumpkin seeds and stir very well in order to coat the seeds
5. Add 1 dollop of pumpkin seeds over a baking sheet; then repeat the same process
6. Bake the pumpkin seeds into the oven for about 18 minutes
7. Remove the pumpkin seeds from the oven and let it cool down for several minutes
8. Once the pumpkin seeds are cool, press several pumpkin seeds with your hands to make clusters
9. Press the clusters very well to avoid falling apart
10. Once the pumpkin clusters are dry and cool; serve and enjoy it with cereal

NURITION

Kcal: 110.5 Fat: 3.2 Carbs: 12 Proteins: 4.2

CAULIFLOWER POPCORN

Prep Time: 10 Minutes| Cooking Time: 30 Minutes| Servings: 3-4

INGREDIENTS

- ½ Medium head of cauliflower
- Extra virgin olive oil
- 1 Pinch of salt
- ½ Teaspoon of onion powder
- ½ Teaspoon of dried chives

DIRECTIONS:

1. Preheat your oven to a temperature of about 450° F
2. Cut the cauliflower into small pieces; then drizzle with with the olive oil
3. Sprinkle the cauliflower with 1 pinch of salt
4. Spread the cauliflower over a baking sheet lined with a parchment paper
5. Bake the cauliflower into the oven for about 30 minutes; make sure to flip the cauliflower at least 2 thrice or twice; otherwise you will risk burning it
6. Remove the cauliflower from the oven and sprinkle with chives and onion powder
7. Serve and enjoy your cauliflower popcorn!

NURITION

Kcal: 105.4 Fat: 1.6 Carbs: 15 Proteins: 11.8

SALAD RECIPES

CABBAGE AND KALE SALAD

Prep Time: 5 Minutes| Cooking Time: 0 Minutes| Servings: 2-3

INGREDIENTS:
- 1 Cup of shredded green cabbage
- ½ Cup of shredded red cabbage
- 2 Cups of shredded raw kale
- 2 Shredded carrots
- 1 Cored, peeled and thinly sliced apple
- ¼ Cup of slivered almonds
- ¼ Cup of fresh blueberries
- ¼ Cup of extra virgin olive oil
- 2 Tablespoons of apple cider vinegar
- 2 Tablespoons of raw honey
- 1 Tablespoon of lemon juice
- 1 Pinch of sea salt
- 1 Pinch of freshly ground black pepper

DIRECTIONS :
1. In a deep salad bowl, combine the green cabbage with the red cabbage, the carrots, the kale, the apple, and the blueberries.
2. Into a small bowl, mix the olive oil, the apple cider vinegar, the honey
3. Add the lemon juice; the salt and the pepper
4. Drizzle your vinaigrette over the salad and toss very well until your ingredients are very well blended
5. Top your salad with slivered almonds
6. Serve and enjoy your salad!

NURITION
Kcal: 317 Fat: 27 Carbs: 13 Proteins: 5.6

LETTUCE SALAD

Prep Time: 5 Minutes| Cooking Time: 0 Minutes| Servings: 3

INGREDIENTS
- ½ Torn green oak lettuce
- ½ Diced avocado
- 1 Large chopped mango
- 2 Tablespoons of toasted slivered almonds
- 2 Tablespoons of dried cranberries
- 1 Tablespoon of olive oil
- 1 Tablespoon of white wine vinegar

DIRECTIONS :
1. Combine the lettuce with the avocado, the mango, the almonds and the cranberries into a deep and large bowl.
2. Whisk the oil and the vinegar altogether in a small bowl
3. Add a pinch of salt and a pinch of pepper.
4. Pour the seasoning over the mixture of the lettuce.
5. Toss the ingredients of the salt very well to combine it
6. Serve and enjoy your salad!

NURITION
Kcal: 373.5 Fat: 19.7 Carbs: 8.9 Proteins: 6

BEET SALAD

Prep Time: 5 Minutes| Cooking Time: 0 Minutes| Servings: 2

INGREDIENTS:
- 2 Large beets, peeled, boiled and chopped
- 1 Small white onion, peeled and chopped
- 1 Medium ripe tomato, finely chopped
- 2 Tablespoons of olive oil
- 2 Tablespoons of fresh and finely chopped Chives and parsley
- 3 Tablespoons of olive oil
- 2 Tablespoons of balsamic vinegar
- 1 Pinch of salt
- 1 Pinch of freshly ground black pepper

DIRECTIONS :
1. Combine the diced avocado, onion, tomato and beets in a large mixing bowl
2. In a separate shallow dish, mix the vinegar with the oil, salt, herbs and pepper
3. Dress your veggies with the vinegar and oil and toss very well
4. Refrigerate the salad for about 1 hour
5. Garnish with chopped chives and flat parsley
6. Serve and enjoy your salad!

NURITION
Kcal: 122.1
Fat: 7.9
Carbs: 9.8
Proteins: 3.7

STRAWBERRY SALAD

Prep Time: 5 Minutes| Cooking Time: 0 Minutes| Servings: 2-3

INGREDIENTS
- 3 cups of torn mixed salad greens
- cups of fresh strawberries, sliced
- 1 package of about 4 ounces of crumbled feta cheese
- ¼ cup of sunflower kernels
- 1 Tablespoon of balsamic vinaigrette

DIRECTIONS
1. Place the first 4 ingredients into a large bowl
2. Mix your ingredients very well
3. Drizzle with the vinaigrette; then toss very well to combine
4. Serve and enjoy your salad!

NURITION
Kcal: 103 Fat: 6 Carbs: 3 Proteins: 6.1

PEA AND BACON SALAD

Prep Time: 5 Minutes| Cooking Time: 0 Minutes| Servings: 3

INGREDIENTS

- 4 cups of frozen peas, about 16 ounces
- ½ cup of shredded sharp cheddar cheese
- ½ cup of ranch salad dressing
- 1/3 cup of chopped red onion
- ¼ teaspoon of salt
- ¼ teaspoon of pepper
- cooked and crumbled bacon strips

DIRECTIONS

1. Combine all of our first 6 ingredients; then toss very well to coat
2. Refrigerate, covered, for about at least 30 minutes
3. Stir in the bacon before serving
4. Serve and enjoy your salad!

NURITION

Kcal: 218 Fat: 14 Carbs: 13 Proteins: 9

STRAWBERRY AND CASHEW SALAD

Prep Time: 5 Minutes| Cooking Time: 0 Minutes| Servings: 2-3

INGREDIENTS

- 4 cups of sliced fresh strawberries
- tablespoons of caramel ice cream topping
- 2 tablespoons of maple syrup
- 1 tablespoon of orange juice
- 1/3 cup of salted cashew halves

DIRECTIONS

1. Place the strawberries into a large bowl
2. Add in the caramel topping, the syrup and orange juice; then drizzle over the strawberries.
3. Top with the cashews.
4. Serve and enjoy your salad

NURITION

Kcal: 116 Fat: 4 Carbs: 20 Proteins: 2

SHREDDED KALE SALAD

Prep Time: 5 Minutes| Cooking Time: 0 Minutes| Servings: 2

INGREDIENTS

- 1 small bunch of kale (about 8 ounces), stemmed as well as thinly sliced
- ½ pound of fresh thinly sliced Brussels sprouts, thinly sliced (about 3 cups)
- ½ cup of coarsely chopped pistachios
- ½ cup of honey mustard salad dressing
- ¼ cup of shredded Parmesan cheese

DIRECTIONS

1. In a large bowl, mix your ingredients
2. Season very well with salt and drizzle with olive oil
3. Top with coarsely chopped ripe pear and cheese
4. Serve and enjoy your salad!

NURITION

Kcal: 207 Fat: 14 Carbs: 16 Proteins: 7

PLUM SALAD

Prep Time: 5 Minutes| Cooking Time: 0 Minutes| Servings: 3

INGREDIENTS

- ½ cup of olive oil
- ½ cup of maple syrup
- ¼ cup or rice vinegar
- tablespoons of Dijon mustard
- ¼ teaspoon of salt
- ¼ teaspoon of pepper

For the SALAD:

- ripe sliced plums
- packages of about 10 ounces each of baby kale salad blend
- 1 cup of pomegranate seeds

DIRECTIONS

1. Put the first 6 ingredients into a jar with a lid; then shake very well
2. Season with the salt
3. Refrigerate the salad until serving
4. To serve your salad, shake the vinaigrette and toss about ½ cup with the persimmons or plumes.
5. Toss the remaining vinaigrette with the salad blend.
6. Top with the persimmons and the pomegranate seeds.
7. Serve and enjoy your salad!

NURITION

Kcal: 175 Fat: 9 Carbs: 23 Proteins: 2

BREAD

SWISS BREAD

Prep Time: 15 Minutes| Cooking Time: 60 Minutes| Servings: 5-6

INGREDIENTS

1. ounces of Jarlsberg or Swiss cheese
2. cups of all-purpose flour
3. tablespoons of sugar
4. teaspoons of baking powder
5. 1 ½ teaspoons of salt
6. ½ teaspoon of pepper
7. 1 bottle of about 12 ounces of beer or of non-alcoholic beer
8. 2 tablespoons of melted butter

DIRECTIONS

- Preheat your oven to about 375°; then divide the cheese into half and cut into cubes of about ¼ in each; then shred the remaining cheese.
- In a bowl, then combine the next 5 ingredients and stir in the beer into your dry ingredients just until everything is moistened
- Fold in the cubed and the shredded cheese.
- Transfer your mixture to a greased loaf pan of about 8x4-in; then drizzle with the butter.
- Bake for about 50 to 60 minutes then cool for 10 minutes
- Slice, then serve and enjoy your bread!

NURITION

Kcal: 182 Fat: 5 Carbs: 28 Proteins: 6

MONKEY BREAD

Prep Time: 10 Minutes| Cooking Time: 22 Minutes| Servings: 6

INGREDIENTS

1. ¼ cup of minced fresh parsley
2. ¼ cup of olive oil
3. 2 tablespoons of minced fresh oregano
4. 1 tablespoon of white wine vinegar
5. 2 Minced garlic cloves
6. ¾ teaspoon of kosher salt
7. ¼ teaspoon of ground cumin
8. ¼ teaspoon of pepper
9. 1/8 teaspoon of crushed red pepper flakes
10. 2 tubes of about 12 ounces each of refrigerated buttermilk biscuits

DIRECTIONS

- In a large shallow bowl, combine all of the first 9 ingredients; then cut each of the biscuits into half and shape into a dough ball
- Roll into the herb mixture.
- Place the biscuit pieces into a greased 10-in. Tube pan of a fluted shape
- Bake at about 375°F for about 18 to 22 minutes
- Slice; then serve and enjoy your bread!

NURITION

Kcal: 209 Fat: 11 Carbs: 25 Proteins: 3

GREEN ONION ROLLS

Prep Time: 20 Minutes| Cooking Time: 20 Minutes| Servings: 5

INGREDIENTS

1. 1 tablespoon of butter
2. 1 and ½ cups of chopped green onions
3. ½ teaspoon of pepper
4. ¾ teaspoon of garlic salt
5. 1 loaf of about 1 pound of frozen bread dough
6. ½ cup of shredded with the part-skim mozzarella cheese
7. 1/3 cup of grated Parmesan cheese

DIRECTIONS

- Preheat your oven to a temperature of about 375°; then in a large skillet, heat the butter over a medium-high heat; then sauté the green onions until they become tender
- Stir in the pepper and if needed the garlic the salt, remove from the heat.
- Over a lightly floured surface, roll the dough into a about 12x8-in rectangular an
- Spread with the onion mixture; sprinkle with the cheeses.
- Roll up the jelly-roll style, starting with the long side; then pinch seam to seal.
- Cut into about 12 slices; then place into some greased muffin cups.
- Cover; then let rise into a warm place for about 30 minutes
- Preheat your oven to about 375°F; then bake for about 18 to 20 minutes
- Serve and enjoy

NURITION

Kcal: 142 Fat: 4 Carbs: 20 Proteins: 6.3

SWEET HONEY BREAD

Prep Time: 10 Minutes| Cooking Time: 30 Minutes| Servings: 4

INGREDIENTS

- 3 Teaspoon of olive oil
- 3 Cups of all purpose flour
- ½ Teaspoon of bicarbonate baking soda
- 1 Teaspoon of salt
- 1 and ¼ cup of whole milk or plain yogurt
- Water
- 3 Tbsp of honey
- 1Tbsp of sugar

DIRECTIONS:

1 Start by preparing your Instant Pot and place the steaming basket inside it. And grease with oil 4 heat proof containers or a tray that fits the Instant Pot.
1. Meanwhile, combine all together, the flour, the baking soda and the salt, then add the sugar and the honey.
2. Mix the ingredients very well together with the help of a fork and after that; add yogurt, and stir very well and add a little bit of water; then knead the ingredients.
3. Form 4 small dough balls. The sough shall be sticky, but not too much.
2 5.   Place every ball in a container or place all the balls into the baking tray and   oil the top or you can brush the top with butter or milk.
4. Cover the containers with foil and make sure they are tightly closed.
5. Lock the lid of the instant pot after lining the containers inside and set at high pressure for 30 minutes.
6. When the timer beeps, naturally release the pressure and let the containers cool for 10 minutes; check with a toothpick and if it comes clean, serve and enjoy your sweet bread!

NURITION

Kcal: 100 Fat: 4 Carbs: 56 Proteins: 2.3

WHOLE-WHEAT FLOUR

Prep Time: 15 Minutes| Cooking Time: 45 Minutes| Servings: 5-6

INGREDIENTS

- 2 cups of all-purpose flour
- 1 cup of white whole-wheat flour
- 1 ¾ teaspoons of salt
- ½ teaspoon of active dry yeast
- 2 tablespoons plus 1 teaspoon of fresh chopped rosemary
- 1 and ½ cups of room temperature water

DIRECTIONS:

1. In a large glass bowl large that fits your Instant Pot, mix all together the salt, the flour, the yeast and 2 tablespoons of fresh rosemary.
2. Pour in the water and combine very well with a spatula or a wooden spoon; but don't over mix
3. Place a trivet into the bottom of your Instant Pot, you need to remove the inner cooking pot
4. Cover the bowl with a plastic wrap; then place the trivet in the Instant Pot and turn on the setting function yogurt; then turn the vent to venting
5. Set the timer for about 4 hours for the dough to proof
6. When your dough is done proofing, preheat your oven to 450°F and place a Dutch oven with cover in the oven to warm up
7. Place the dough over a floured counter and shape into a dough
8. Brush the dough with olive oil and sprinkle with sea salt and with the remaining rosemary.
9. Let stand aside; then remove the hot Dutch oven from your oven and uncover it
10. Put the dough ball in your Dutch oven; then cover it
11. Place back in the oven and cook for about 30 minutes
12. Remove the lid and bake for about 15 additional minutes
13. Remove the bread from the oven and let cool before slicing
14. Serve and enjoy your bread!

NURITION

Kcal: 133 Fat: 0.6 Carbs: 27.9 Proteins: 4.3

BANANA BREAD

Prep Time: 15 Minutes| Cooking Time: 50 Minutes| Servings: 5

INGREDIENTS

- 2 Cups of low carb baking mix
- 2 to 3 medium, fully ripe and mashed bananas
- 2 Tablespoons of butter room temperature
- 2 Large eggs
- 1/3 Cup of unsweetened apple sauce
- ¼ Cup of sugar
- ¼ Cup of chopped nuts
- 1 and ½ teaspoons of baking soda
- ½ Teaspoon of salt

DIRECTIONS:

1. Mix the sugar, the softened butter, the unsweetened applesauce and the eggs
2. With a hand mixer, beat your ingredients very well until it becomes smooth
3. Add the unsweetened applesauce and the eggs
4. Beat your mixture very well until it is very well mixed
5. Add in the mashed bananas to your wet ingredients; then fully mix.
6. Add your dry ingredients to your wet ingredients and whisk very well until your ingredients are combined
7. Add in the nuts; then grease a medium loaf baking tray
8. Pour the mixture into the tray; then cover it with an aluminum foil
9. Pour 1 cup of water into your Instant Pot; then place the trivet in its place
10. Put the baking tray over the trivet and make a shape of handle with the aluminum
11. Lock the lid of the Instant Pot and set the timer on the setting Manual for about 50 minutes
12. When the timer beeps; naturally release the pressure after 10 minutes; then remove the baking tray from the Instant Pot
13. Set the bread aside to cool
14. Slice the bread; then serve and enjoy it!

NURITION

Kcal: 247 Fat: 8.8 Carbs: 39 Proteins: 3.8

APPLE BREAD

Prep Time: 15 Minutes| Cooking Time: 70 Minutes| Servings: 5

INGREDIENTS

- 3 Cups of cubed and peeled apple
- 1 cup of sugar
- 2 large eggs
- 1 tbsp of vanilla
- 1 tbsp of apple pie spice
- 2 cup of flour
- 1 tbsp of butter
- 1 tbsp of baking powder

DIRECTIONS:

1. Mix the eggs, the butter, the cream, the sugar and the pie sauce with a mixer
2. Mix until you get a fluffy and velvety texture; then add the apples into the creamy mixture
3. Mix the flour and the baking powder
4. Add the mixture to the creamy mixture; then pour the batter into the pan and place the pan over the trivet in your Instant Pot
5. Add 1 cup of water to your Instant Pot
6. Set your Instant Pot to "Manual" at High pressure for about 70 minutes
7. Do a quick release pressure method
8. Top with the icing; then serve and enjoy your bread!

NURITION

Kcal: 123.3 Fat: 1 Carbs: 26.4 Proteins: 2.1

SIMPLE BUTTER BREAD

Prep Time: 15 Minutes| Cooking Time: 20 Minutes| Servings: 4

INGREDIENTS

- ½ Pound of wheat flour
- ¼ Cup of sugar
- 1 cup of warm fresh milk
- 1 cup of butter
- 1/3 of an egg
- 1 tbsp of yeast
- ½ tbsp of salt

DIRECTIONS:

1. Combine your ingredients all together except for the butter. Keep mixing your components on a hard surface like marble and use the palms of your hand to make it smooth.
2. Add the butter and blend the mixture very well.
3. Let the bread dough rest for around 2 to 3 hours or until you notice its size double: Make sure to put it in a plastic container or a bag.
4. Tips: Ensure that there is no wind as this may dry up the dough. Also, the longer you proof the bread, the softer it will be - so no shortcuts! Nevertheless, a warmer kitchen can help to speed up the time needed for the proofing.
5. Now, divide your obtained dough into small balls of 30g each.
6. Prepare an egg wash by combining the egg of a yolk with 1 tbsp of milk.
7. With your hands, shape every ball and the place the number of balls you obtain just in one baking paper.
8. Add the pumpkin seeds on top of the dough or you can use sesame too.
9. Brush your balls with the egg wash that you have already prepared.
10. Now, all that is left to do is to let the dough rest again for 30 minutes.
11. Pour 1 ½ cups of water into your Instant Pot
12. Place a trivet in the bottom of your Instant Pot; then Place your dough balls in a sprayed tray and cover with an aluminum foil
13. Close the lid of your Instant Pot and set seal the valve
14. Set the timer for about 20 minutes and pressure cook the bread
15. When the pressure cooking is done, do a quick pressure release method; then when it is safe to do, open the Instant Pot and remove the baking tray
16. Serve and enjoy your bread!

NURITION

Kcal: 252 Fat: 7.4 Carbs: 45 Proteins: 2.8

CRANBERRY BREAD

Prep Time: 20 Minutes| Cooking Time: 45 Minutes| Servings: 5

INGREDIENTS

- 2 ¼ cups of white whole wheat flour
- 1 cup of white flour
- 1 ½ teaspoons of salt
- 1 teaspoon of instant yeast
-
- 1 ½ cups of room temperature water
- ½ cup of pecans, whole and chopped
- ½ cup of cranberries

DIRECTIONS:

1. In a large bowl, mix together the whole-wheat with the white flour, the salt, and the yeast.
2. Add in the water and with your bare hands, combine until you get an incorporated dough; if the dough is sticky; sprinkle 2 tablespoons of flour on top and fold it
3. Place the dough on a parchment paper; then put inside your Instant pot liner
4. Lock the lid of the Instant Pot and seal the valve
5. Press the setting function yogurt, then adjust until you see the display 24:00 and adjust the timer to 4:30
6. Wait for the beeper to indicate that the cycle has started and after about 4 hours
7. Grab the sides of the parchment paper to lift the dough; then pat the dough into a rectangular shape and sprinkle with the cranberries and the pecans
8. Pull the edges of your dough on top of the cranberries and pecans
9. Place back into the center of the parchment paper; then in your Instant Pot and secure the lid
10. Place a 6 to 8 cast iron pot in your oven with the lid on
11. Preheat your oven to 450°F and after about 30 minutes, remove the pot from the oven and place the lid to the side
12. Lift the dough from the pot and place it in the cast iron pot and put inside the oven
13. Bake for about 30 minutes
14. Remove the lid of the pot; then bake for about 15 additional minutes
15. Remove from the oven; then hold the corners of the paper very well
16. Place the bread over a cooling rack; then serve and enjoy your bread!

NURITION

Kcal: 252 Fat: 4 Carbs: 36.2 Proteins: 5.5

CHEDDAR CHEESE BREAD

Prep Time: 20 Minutes| Cooking Time: 55 Minutes| Servings: 5

INGREDIENTS
- 1 bottle of beer
- 3 cups of self rising flour
- 2 tbsp of melted salted butter
- 1 can of diced chiles optional, about 4 oz.
- ½ cup of shredded cheddar cheese

DIRECTIONS:
1. In a large bowl; pour a bottle of beer in; then gently mix with the flour
2. Pour in the melted butter and gently fold in
3. Spray a pan with non stick cooking spray
4. Pour the beer bread mixture in; then cover with a paper towel; then a tinfoil
5. Pour 2 cups of water in your Instant Pot pressure cooker; then put a trivet in
6. Lower the pan on the trivet and close the lid of the Instant Pot
7. Seal the valve and set the pressure cooking time to about 55 minutes at High pressure
8. Allow the pressure to naturally release
9. Flip the bread to a cutting board; then cut into pieces
10. Serve and enjoy the bread with dip of your choice!

NURITION
Kcal: 171 Fat: 5 Carbs: 24 Proteins: 5

CHOCOLATE BREAD

Prep Time: 20 Minutes| Cooking Time: 60 Minutes| Servings: 4

INGREDIENTS
- ¾ cup of whole wheat flour
- ¾ cup of white flour
- ½ tsp of baking powder
- 1 tsp of baking soda
- 1/3 cup of brown sugar
- 1/3 cup of white sugar
- ½ tsp of salt
- 1 Large egg
- ½ cup of oil
- 2 Small, peeled and mashed ripe bananas
- 1 Shredded small zucchini
- 1 cup of semi sweet mini chocolate chips
- 1 cup of water

DIRECTIONS:
1. Grease a 6-cups Bundt pan and keep it aside.
2. In a large bowl, mix all together the flours, the sugars, the baking powder, the baking soda and the salt.
3. In a separate bowl, add the egg, the oil and the banana and beat until very well combined.
4. Add the flour mixture; then mix very well until your ingredients are very well combined
5. Gently, add in the chocolate chips and the zucchini
6. Place your mixture into the prepared pan; then with a piece of foil, cover the top of your pan.
7. Place a steamer trivet in the bottom of your Instant Pot and pour in the water.
8. Put the pan over the trivet; then secure the lid and turn to "Sealed" position
9. Cook on "Manual" with a "High Pressure" For about 60 minutes
10. Press the button "Cancel"; then do a natural release method
11. Remove the lid of your Instant Pot; then transfer the pan to a wire rack and let cool for about 10 minutes
12. Invert the bread and cut into slices; then serve and enjoy the bread!

NURITION
Kcal: 122 Fat: 2 Carbs: 24 Proteins: 3

DESERTS

SESAME CRACKERS

Prep Time: 10 Minutes| Cooking Time: 18 Minutes| Servings: 9

INGREDIENTS:

- ½ Cup of almond meal
- 1/3 Cup of sesame seeds
- 1 Teaspoon of olive oil
- 1 Large egg white
- 1 Pinch of salt
- 1 Pinch of fresh ground black pepper

DIRECTIONS :

1. Preheat your oven to a temperature of about 365° F.
2. Put all the ingredients into a large bowl and mix very well
3. Put the mixture over a baking sheet; then cover it with another baking sheet
4. Roll the mixture with a rolling pin
5. Score the pastry with the back of your knife into pieces shaped into squares
6. Remove the baking paper from the top of your pastry and transfer it to a baking pan
7. Put the pastry in the oven for about 18 minutes
8. Serve and enjoy!

NURITION

Kcal: 148.5 Fat: 12 Carbs: 3.3 Proteins: 7.2

PEACH COBBLER

Prep Time: 10 Minutes| Cooking Time: 25 Minutes| Servings: 3

INGREDIENTS:

- 1 Cup of dried peaches
- 1 Cup of roasted almonds
- ½ Cup of shredded unsweetened coconut
- 1 Tablespoon of olive oil
- 1 Large egg

DIRECTIONS :

1. Put the peaches, the almonds and the coconut into a food processor and pulse it
2. Drizzle in the olive oil and pulse for a few more seconds
3. In a large mixing bowl, combine the mixture with the egg and whisk very well
4. Make about patties by rolling it; then press the dough and arrange the patties over a baking sheet
5. Bake your patties in the oven at a temperature of about 350°F for about 25 minutes
6. Serve and enjoy your peach bites!

NURITION

Kcal: 120 Fat: 7.8 Carbs: 14 Proteins: 34.9

COCOA BALLS

Prep Time: 10 Minutes| Cooking Time: 0 Minutes| Servings: 6

INGREDIENTS

- 2 tablespoons of raw cocoa
- 3 tablespoons of flaxseed oatmeal
- 2 cups of peanut almond butter
- 1 Tablespoon of organic chia seeds
- 2 Tablespoons of Protein powder

DIRECTIONS :

1. Mix the raw cacao, oatmeal, 3 tablespoons of the protein powder, peanut butter and 1 tablespoon of chia seed.
2. Form balls
3. Roll in raw cocoa.
4. Put in the fridge 1 hour
5. Serve and enjoy your dessert!

NURITION

Kcal: 388 Fat: 33.7 Carbs: 7 Proteins: 7.5

COCONUT GINGER PATTIES

Prep Time: 10 Minutes| Cooking Time: 0 Minutes| Servings: 7

INGREDIENTS:

- 1 ½ Cups of butter, softened
- ½ Cup of shredded coconut; unsweetened
- 1 Teaspoon of Erythritol
- 1 Teaspoon of ginger powder

DIECTIONS :

1. Combine the softened butter with the erythritol, the shredded coconut and the ginger powder and mix very well until your ingredients are very well dissolved
2. Pour the batter into the silicone moulds
3. Refrigerate for about 10 minutes
4. Serve and enjoy your ginger patties!

NURITION

Kcal: 123 Fat: 12.7 Carbs: 2.4 Proteins: 3

BLUEBERRY BOMBS

Prep Time: 10 Minutes| Cooking Time: 0 Minutes| Servings: 8

INGREDIENTS:

- 4 Oz of soft goat cheese
- ½ Cup of fresh blueberries
- 1 Cup of all purpose flour
- 1 Teaspoon of vanilla extract
- ½ Cup of pecans
- ½ Teaspoon of stevia
- ¼ Cup of unsweetened shredded coconut

DIRECTIONS :

1. Process the goat cheese with the fresh blueberries, the flour, the vanilla extract, the pecans, the stevia and the unsweetened shredded coconut in a food processor and process very well
2. Roll the mixture into about 30 small fat bombs
3. Pour the coconut flakes in a bowl
4. Lightly roll each of the fat bombs into the shredded coconut
5. Serve and enjoy your delicious fat bombs!

NURITION

Kcal: 137.1 Fat: 14.3 Carbs: 0.9 Proteins: 2

PEAR CAKE

Prep Time: 10 Minutes| Cooking Time: 0 Minutes| Servings: 8

INGREDIENTS:

- 1 can of about 15 ounces of reduced-sugar sliced pears
- 1 package of white cake mix of a regular size
- 2 to 3 large egg whites, to the room temperature
- 1 large egg to the room temperature
- 2 teaspoons of confectioners' sugar

DIRECTIONS:

1 Drain the pears making sure to reserve the syrup; then chop the pears. Place the pears and the syrup in a bowl; then add in the cake mix, the egg whites and the egg.
2 Beat your ingredients on a low speed for about 30 seconds: then beat on a high speed for about 4 minutes.
3 Coat a fluted tube pan of about 10-in with cooking spray and dust it with the flour; then add in the batter
4 Bake at about 350° for about 50 to 55 minutes; then let cool for about 5 minutes
5 Serve and enjoy your cake!

NURITION

Kcal: 149 Fat: 3 Carbs: 28 Proteins: 2

COCONUT MACAROONS

Prep Time: 10 Minutes| Cooking Time: 20 Minutes| Servings: 7

INGREDIENTS

- 1 and 1/3 cups of sweetened shredded coconut
- 1/3 cup sugar
- 2 tablespoons all-purpose flour
- 1/8 teaspoon salt
- 2 large egg whites, room temperature
- 1/2 teaspoon vanilla extract

DIRECTIONS

1 In a medium bowl, combine all together the coconut with the sugar, the flour and the salt.
2 Add the egg whites and the vanilla; and mix very well.
3 Drop by some rounded teaspoonfuls over some greased baking sheets.
4 Bake at a temperature of about 325°F for about 18 to20 minutes or until your ingredients get a golden brown color
5 Let cool on a wire rack; then serve and enjoy!

NURITION

Kcal: 149 Fat: 3 Carbs: 28 Proteins: 2

CHOCOLATE FONDUE

Prep Time: 10 Minutes| Cooking Time: 2 Hours| Servings: 2-4

INGREDIENTS

- 18 Oz of semisweet chopped chocolate
- 1 Oz of unsweetened chopped chocolate
- 6 Oz of chopped 75% dark chocolate
- 1Can of 13 oz of milk
- 1 Teaspoon of vanilla
- Fruit cookies

DIRECTIONS:

1. Combine the chocolates with the milk into a 3 quart slow cooker
2. Cover your slow cooker with a lid and cook on Low for about 1 to 2 hours
3. When the time is up; turn off your slow cooker; stir very well
4. Add the vanilla and stir
5. Serve and enjoy your dessert!

NURITION

Kcal: 165 Fat: 6.4 Carbs: 10.3 Proteins: 2.6

CHOCOLATE FUDGES

Prep Time: 10 Minutes| Cooking Time: 3 Hours| Servings: 3

INGREDIENTS

- 2 and ½ cups of chocolate chips
- ½ Cup of milk
- 1/8 Teaspoon of sea salt
- 1 Teaspoon of vanilla extract

DIRECTIONS:

1. Grease your slow cooker with oil
2. Pour the coconut milk in a bowl and stir it very well
3. Pour 1 cup of milk in the bottom of your slow cooker and add the remaining ingredients except for the vanilla extract
4. Cover your slow cooker with a lid and cook on High for about 2 hours
5. Add the vanilla; then stir and whisk very well
6. Leave the mixture uncovered for about 3 to 4 hours
7. Serve and enjoy your dessert!

NURITION

Kcal: 160 Fat: 10 Carbs: 11 Proteins: 3

SMOOTHIE

AVOCADO SMOOTHIE

Prep Time: 5 Minutes| Cooking Time: 0 Minutes| Servings: 2

INGREDIENTS:

- 1 ripe avocado peeled and pit removed
- 1 1/3 cup water
- 2-3 tablespoons lemon juice
- 2 Tbsp low carb sugar substitute I like to use 1/8 teaspoon liquid stevia extract
- 1/2 cup frozen unsweetened raspberries or other low carb frozen berries

DIRECTIONS :

1. Add all your ingredients to a blender.
2. Blend your ingredients until it becomes smooth
3. Pour the smoothie into two glasses
4. Serve and enjoy your smoothie!

NURITION

Kcal: 227 Fat: 6 Carbs: 12 Proteins: 2.5

COFFEE SHAKE

Prep Time: 5 Minutes| Cooking Time: 5 Minutes| Servings: 2-3

INGREDIENTS:

- 1 and ½ teaspoons of Sukrin Gold Fiber Syrup
- ½ Teaspoon of Sukrin Gold
- 1 Tablespoon of heavy cream
- ¼ Teaspoon of ground ginger
- 1/8 Teaspoon of ground cinnamon
- 1 Cup of hot brewed coffee
- ¼ Cup of whipped cream
- 1 Dash of ground cloves

DIRECTIONS :

1. Mix all together the sweeteners, the heavy cream, the ginger, and cinnamon in large mug.
2. Add 1 cup of hot brewed coffee.
3. Stir until spices have been blended into coffee.
4. Top with whipped cream and then sprinkle cloves on top

NURITION

Kcal: 453.6 Fat: 37.5 Carbs: 16.8 Proteins: 15.6

RASPBERRY LEMONADE SMOOTHIE

Prep Time: 5 Minutes| Cooking Time: 0 Minutes| Servings: 2

INGREDIENTS:

- 1 Can of chilled Raspberry Lemonade
- ½ Cup of frozen unsweetened fresh raspberries
- ½ Cup of crushed ice
- The juice from one medium lime
- 1/8 Teaspoon of vanilla stevia drops; about 20 drops

DIRECTIONS :

1. Pour all your ingredients into the blender and blend it very well until all your ingredients are very well combined
2. Divide the smoothie into two glasses
3. Serve and enjoy your smoothie!

NURITION

Kcal: 22 Fat: 37.5 Carbs: 5.5 Proteins: 11.5

STRAWBERRY AND KIWI SMOOTHIE

Prep Time: 5 Minutes| Cooking Time: 0 Minutes| Servings: 2-3

INGREDIENTS
- 1 and ½ cups of frozen roughly chopped strawberries
- 1 and ½ cup of roughly chopped frozen kiwi
- 8 Leaves of fresh mint
- 2 Oz of rum
- 2 Cups of crushed ice

DIRECTIONS:
1. Mix the frozen strawberries with about 4 mint leaves
2. Add 1 oz of rum; 1 cup of ice; then blend the ingredients until it becomes smooth into a blender.
3. Pour the strawberry smoothie into glasses
4. Repeat the same process with the kiwis; then pour the strawberry mixture on top
5. Garnish with the fresh strawberries and the mint leaves.
6. Refrigerate your smoothie cold

NURITION
Kcal: 180.2 Fat: 1.7 Carbs: 44.2 Proteins: 2.1

AVOCADO CUCUMBER SMOOTHIE

Prep Time: 5 Minutes| Cooking Time: 0 Minutes| Servings: 2-3

INGREDIENTS:
- 1 Cup of filtered water
- ½ Avocado
- 1 Tablespoon of avocado oil
- ½ Organic Cucumbers
- 1 Handful of dark leafy greens
- 1 to 2 leaves of dandelion
- 2 Tablespoons of parsley
- 2 Tablespoons of hemp seeds
- The juice of 1 lemon
- ¼ Teaspoon of turmeric powder

DIRECTIONS :
1. Blend all your ingredients into a high-speed blender
2. Blend until you get a smooth mixture for about 1 minute
3. Serve and enjoy your delicious smoothie!

NURITION
Kcal: 360 Fat: 3 Carbs: 8 Proteins: 10

STRAWBERRY SMOOTHIE

Prep Time: 5 Minutes| Cooking Time: 0 Minutes| Servings: 3

INGREDIENTS:
- 5 to 6 Whole frozen strawberries
- 2 Scoops of unflavored whey protein; about 2/3 cup
- 2 and ½ cups of milk
- 1 Teaspoon of vanilla extract
- 2 Packets of stevia

DIRECTIONS :
1. Place the strawberries, the protein mixture, the milk, the vanilla, and the sugar substitute in a blender
2. Blend your ingredients at a high speed until you get a smooth mixture
3. Add some ice to add extra cold if you want it cold
4. Serve and enjoy your dish!

NURITION
Kcal: 187 Fat: 4 Carbs: 5 Proteins: 26

SPINACH AND PEPPER MINT SMOOTHIE

Prep Time: 5 Minutes| Cooking Time: 0 Minutes| Servings: 2-3

INGREDIENTS

- ½ avocado
- 1 Cup of fresh spinach
- 10 to 12 drops Liquid Stevia Peppermint Sweet Drops
- 1 Scoop of whey protein powder
- ½ Cup of milk
- ¼ Teaspoon of peppermint extract
- 1 Cup of ice
- Optional ingredients: Cacao nibs

DIRECTIONS :

1. Place the avocado, the spinach, the protein powder and the milk in a blender
2. Blend your mixture until it becomes smooth
3. Add in the stevia peppermint Sweet Drops, the extract, and the ice, and blend very well
4. Taste the smoothie
5. Serve and enjoy your delicious smoothie!

NURITION

Kcal: 293 Fat: 11 Carbs: 8 Proteins: 28

BLUEBERRY AND LEMON SMOOTHIE

Prep Time: 5 Minutes| Cooking Time: 0 Minutes| Servings: 2

INGREDIENTS

- ¼ Cup of heavy whipping cream
- ¾ Cup of milk
- 2 Ounces of cream cheese
- 2 Teaspoons of granulated stevia/erythritol blend or sugar
- 1/3 Cup of frozen blueberries
- 1 Scoop of collagen peptides
- ½ Cup of ice
- ½Teaspoon of vanilla extract
- 1 to 5 Drops of lemon extract

DIRECTIONS :

1. Place all your ingredients in a blender.
2. Close the lid of the blender and blend until the ice and the berries are crushed very well
3. Pour the smoothie into 2 glasses
4. Serve and enjoy your delicious smoothie!

NURITION

Kcal: 251 Fat: 22 Carbs: 6 Proteins: 8

AVOCADO AND MANGO SMOOTHIE

Prep Time: 5 Minutes| Cooking Time: 0 Minutes| Servings: 2

INGREDIENTS:

- 2 Ripe peeled and pitted avocados
- 2 Cup of water
- 6 Tablespoons of fresh lemon juice
- 2 Tablespoons of sugar
- 2/3 Cup of fresh or frozen mango

DIRECTIONS :

1. Peel and pit a mango; then slice it into small chunks
2. Peel and pit the avocados and slice into small chunks.
3. Mix the water, the avocado, the lemon juice, the sugar substitute and the mango in a blender
4. Blend all your ingredients for about 30 seconds or just until it reaches the consistency you are looking for
5. Pour the smoothie into two clean glasses and garnish with mango slices
6. Serve and enjoy!

NURITION

Kcal: 341 Fat: 30 Carbs: 22 Proteins: 8

PINEAPPLE AND PARSLEY SMOOTHIE

Prep Time: 5 Minutes| Cooking Time: 0 Minutes| Servings: 3

INGREDIENTS:

- 1 ½ Cups of water or of milk
- 1 Cup of kale chopped
- ¼ Cup of pineapple frozen
- 1 Tablespoon of mint or of parsley
- ½ Tablespoon of peeled fresh ginger fresh
- ½ avocado

DIRECTIONS :

1. Place your ingredients in a blender
2. Blend all your ingredients in a high-powered smoothie blender and puree the mixture until it becomes smooth
3. Start with about 1 cup of liquid; then add in more liquid
4. Serve and enjoy your delicious smoothie!

NURITION

Kcal: 229 Fat: 15 Carbs: 21 Proteins: 5

APPLE SMOOTHIE

Prep Time: 5 Minutes| Cooking Time: 0 Minutes| Servings: 2

INGREDIENTS:

- 1 Medium chopped Apple
- ½ Cup of Heavy cream
- 5 oz of Cream Cheese
- ½ Cup of Milk
- ¼ Cup of Almonds

DIRECTIONS :

1. Place the heavy cream, the milk and the apple in a blender
2. Blend your ingredients for about 3 to 4 minutes
3. Once you get a smooth mixture; add in the cream cheese and the milk
4. Blend your mixture for about 5 additional minutes
5. Pour the smoothie into glasses; then serve and enjoy it!

NURITION

Kcal: 227 Fat: 19 Carbs: 10 Proteins: 7.1

Weekly MEAL PLAN 16:8

	BREAKFAST	SNACK	LUNCH	DINNER
M	Two whole-wheat toasts with red fruit jam, coffee and Greek yogurt.	15 grams of dried fruit rather than 50 grams of rice cakes.	Whole wheat pasta with meat sauce, grilled eggplant and a seasonal fruit.	Baked cod, pan-seared zucchini with extra virgin olive oil and a seasonal fruit.
T	4 dry cookies and 1 cup of semi-skimmed milk.	Avocado toast or 15 grams of walnuts.	Whole wheat pasta with pesto, baked pumpkin cubes and a fresh fruit.	Salmon fillet flavored with lime and sweet paprika, iceberg salad with extra virgin olive oil and one fresh fruit.
W	slices of toast with orange marmalade and a pot of low-fat, sugar-free yogurt.	A seasonal fruit.	Rice with tomato sauce, mixed seasonal vegetables in a pan and a fresh fruit.	Chicken breast cooked in a pan, baked peppers with extra virgin olive oil and a seasonal fruit.
T	Corn flakes with a cup of semi-skimmed milk.	Red fruit salad with Greek yogurt.	Caprese with mozzarella cheese, fresh tomato and basil, chicken breast and a seasonal fruit.	Smoked salmon, mashed potatoes without butter but with extra virgin olive oil, a seasonal fruit.
F	4 slices of toast, red fruit jam and 1 pot of yogurt.	Greek yogurt with honey and walnuts.	Whole-wheat or legume pasta with pesto, fresh salad and 1 fresh fruit in season.	Cod or sea bass in a baked crust, grilled zucchini with extra virgin olive oil and a fresh fruit.
S	Greek yogurt with walnuts and corn muesli.	15 grams of walnuts or hazelnuts.	Saffron rice without butter, pan-seared trevisana salad and one piece of fruit.	Salmon with spices and citrus in a pan, baked potatoes and 1 fresh seasonal fruit.
S	4 slices of whole wheat bread with citrus or apricot jam.	1 slice of banana bread without butter but with extra virgin olive oil.	Whole-wheat pasta with diced ham, fried zucchini and 1 fresh fruit.	Grilled chicken breast, baked peppers with extra virgin olive oil and 1 fresh fruit in season.

Weekly MEAL PLAN 16:8

	BREAKFAST	SNACK	LUNCH	DINNER
M	2 hardboiled eggs + 100 grams of oatmeal and water	1 apple	Salad made of tuna, cherry tomatoes and avocado	1 white chicken breast with steamed broccoli
T	Protein shake and berries	20 gr dried almonds	1 cup of rice with grilled fish	Spinach salad with turkey breast and second green vegetable of choice
W	1 slice of whole wheat banana bread + 1 cup of orange juice	Protein shake	Whole wheat pasta with tomatoes sauce and one spoon of grated cheese	Lettuce, tomatoes, fresh diced cucumber and one can of tuna without oil
T	2 scrambled egg and smoked salmon	10 baby carrots and hummus	Grilled chicken breast, with avocado and lettuce salad	1 portion of brown rice with tofu, grilled vegetables of choice
F	100 gm of oatmeal with milk, scoop of peanut butter	Protein shake	Whole wheat pasta with pesto and 50 gr of bread	Grilled fish, 100gr boiled potatoes
S	1 hardboiled egg, 1 slice of whole wheat bread, avocado	1 bowl of fruits	Chicken grilled salad wrap	1 bowl of mixed vegetables soup, 1 slice of whole wheat bread
S	Protein shake and berries	20 gr dried almonds	Lettuce, raw mushroom, cherry tomatoes, and mozzarella salad	Cauliflower crust vegetarian pizza

Weekly MEAL PLAN 16:8

	BREAKFAST	SNACK	LUNCH	DINNER
M	3 hardboiled eggs, protein shake	10 baby carrots and hummus	Mozzarella, cherry tomatoes, avocado salad	Grilled fish, steamed green vegetables
T	1 whole wheat toast bread, 1 spoon peanut butter	5 slices of deli wrapped with 2 slices of choice of cheese	Spaghetti squash with ragù sauce	Oven shrimps, grilled zucchini
W	2 egg scrambled, smoked salmon slice	Protein shake of choice	2 slices whole bread, choice of dressing, turkey breast deli, 1 slice of choice of cheese	Tofu, vegetables, brown rice
T	Dried fruits	Cheese, cracker, strawberry	Smoked tilapia, green beans	Bowl of mixed vegetable soup
F	1 hardboiled egg, 1 slice of whole meat bread toast, 1 spoon of peanut butter	Rice cake, half banana, Greek yogurt	Turkey sausage, grilled broccoli, grilled pepper	Lettuce, cherry tomatoes, grilled shrimp
S	Protein shake	10 baby carrots and humus	Grilled chicken breast, lettuce, avocado	Grilled salmon, oven asparagus
S	100 gr oatmeal with water, berries	Zero fat Greek yogurt, berries	Chicken and vegetable wrap	Oven tilapia, oven potatoes

CONCLUSION

Intermittent fasting is an eating habit characterized by frequent, brief fasts. Regular 14 to 16-hour fasts, the 5:2 plan, or adapted alternate-day fasting are the safest for women.

A significant component of intermittent fasting's effectiveness is developing an awareness of food intake. You may find it easy to eliminate harmful ingredients such as refined carbohydrates, empty calories, and fats. Merging intermittent fasting for other diets often contributes to the diet's effectiveness.

Although intermittent fasting has been shown to benefit weight loss, diabetes, and heart health, some research suggests that it can have a detrimental impact on some women's blood glucose levels and fertility. Having said that, adapted forms of intermittent fasting tend to be healthy for many women and could be a better choice than longer or more rigorous fasts. To minimize side effects, women should practice gentle fasting, with fewer fasting days and shorter fasts.

If you are a woman trying to lose weight or enhance your fitness, you should certainly try intermittent fasting. Women can benefit from intermittent fasting by losing weight and lowering their risk of diabetes and heart disease. Additional human trials, however, are needed to validate these results.

Exercise when fasting is not just permissible, and it is highly beneficial for hormonal enhancement (which is critical for a variety of health benefits, particularly improved body composition). You can increase the effectiveness of intermittent fasting and burst training by mixing both for a multi-restorative strategy. Weight and cardio training can both be performed when fasting, but you should consult a physician first.

Made in the USA
Las Vegas, NV
02 July 2022